# CONSTRUCTING
# THE
# CROSSFIT GAMES

- DAVE CASTRO -

# CONSTRUCTING THE CROSSFIT GAMES

DAVE CASTRO

PUBLISHED BY
CrossFit, Inc.
1500 Green Hills Road
Scotts Valley, CA, USA

ACKNOWLEDGEMENTS
Editor: Mike Warkentin

Copy Editor: Brittney Saline

Typeset and Cover Design: Susannah Dy

Library of Congress Cataloging-in-Publication Data Pending

ISBN: 978-0-9986150-5-9

Printed in the USA

# TABLE *of* CONTENTS

# PREFACE

*Tuesday, Sept. 5, 12:35 p.m.*

The 2017 Reebok CrossFit Games concluded a month ago in Madison, Wisconsin.

For four days in August, Tia-Clair Toomey from Australia and Mat Fraser from the United States battled the best athletes in the world to be crowned champions of the CrossFit Games.

We make this claim based on their performance. Mat finished first and Tia-Clair finished 18th among 380,000 Open participants. Mat dominated the East Regional, and Tia-Clair finished second in the Pacific Regional to earn their spots in the Games.

At the Games, we test the best of the best and name one man and one woman the Fittest on Earth. In 2017, the Games started on Thursday, Aug. 3, with three separate events. The athletes faced four events on Friday, three on Saturday and three on Sunday—13 scored challenges over four consecutive days of competition.

These events allow the fittest man and woman alive to prove themselves among their rivals and earn the right to stand above them on the podium. I believe it's important to demonstrate that this process is not simply a matter of jotting down some movements on a piece of a paper and then having the athletes do them. Nor is it random, although we believe the best athletes are prepared for any physical challenge. This principle is part of our DNA, and we created the first event of the 2007 CrossFit Games by randomly drawing from a hopper, but the Games are far from random.

The purpose of this book is to chronicle the process I used to develop and refine the events that test the Fittest on Earth. I'm going to take you from the early stages of the season to the end of the CrossFit Games, and I'll share detailed thoughts on every aspect of the competition. I'll cover the entire 2017 season, including the workouts of the Open and Regional rounds that narrowed the field for the premier competition in Madison.

The process I'm going to describe was unique to the 2017 season, and it will likely be different in future years.

But in 2017, this is how I manufactured the tests that defined the CrossFit Games and determined the Fittest on Earth.

# APRIL 2017

*Thursday, April 6, 10:23 a.m.*

Programming the CrossFit Games is hard. I place a lot of pressure on myself to make the event the spectacle that it is. I do not take the job of finding the world's fittest man and woman lightly. I strive to make it the best competition it can be, year after year.

The drive to make it great is part of who I am: I want to be great at everything. I want to succeed, excel and perform at a high level. This started in my childhood and continued into my 20s, years I spent in the U.S. Navy.

Pursuing excellence wasn't a choice but a requirement in the organizations I joined. I'll talk more about my time in the Navy later. Or, more accurately, I'll talk about why I won't talk about the time I spent in the Navy. Suffice it to say that conditions necessitated excellence. Being great, being the best at everything, was all I knew. It was a way of life. It was how I was brought up. If you were not the best or did not strive to be the best, you would be replaced or marginalized, and I would never settle for a spot in the back of the pack.

After 12 years in the Navy, I got out to work full time for CrossFit Inc. As I write these words, I have been working for CrossFit for 11 years, and I'm seven years out of the Navy. I'm currently on our company's twin-turboprop plane, flying to a meeting at our office in Scotts Valley, California, from my home in Carlsbad.

We just flew over Los Angeles, and Dodger Stadium was visible from my seat. I was daydreaming, and an idea just came to me. I've long wanted to write about the history of the CrossFit Games but had no idea how I would ever do it. Writing a complete history of a decade of the CrossFit Games is not something I have time for. But then I thought of Lil Wayne's book, "*Gone 'Til November*," a series of journal entries chronicling his time spent on Rikers Island.

"*That's it*," I realized. My book will be about the 2017 Games as seen through my experience. So the book starts now, April 6, 2017, 11,000 feet over Los Angeles on a private plane. Yes, that's right: a Lil Wayne book is inspiring me to write this.

The meeting I'm flying to attend with other CrossFit HQ staff has nothing to do with the Games. I am not thinking about this meeting. I'm thinking about programming the 2017 Reebok CrossFit Games, and it's stressing me out. The meeting is actually a hassle for me, an annoyance at this stage. We're five months out from the Games, and the programming phase begins now.

This is my 11th year of programming the CrossFit Games. The annual competition started as a small gathering in 2007 on my parents' Northern California ranch. I organized and programmed the early years of the Games, and I continue to program them a decade later. As the event has grown in scale, so has the amount of time and energy I put into it.

At this point, I'm finished with the programming for the second phase of qualification: Regionals. I completed the task yesterday, to be exact. Now I have to dive into the Games planning.

I often say that I plan and program the Games year round, and that I plan years in advance. This is true. For example, I knew the Games would return to The Ranch at some point three or four years before it happened in 2016. I thought about the return and planned for it during the years leading up to the 10th edition of the Games, the last to be held in Carson, California.

For this year's Games in Madison, I have new ideas, plans and concepts I have been thinking about since I scouted Madison in September 2016.

Madison has been a breath of fresh air for me. Those closest to me and the process knew that the canvas of Carson was getting tired for me. Planning at the same venue for seven years was becoming stale and boring. I wouldn't say the venue negatively affected anything we did there, but staying at the StubHub Center in Carson would likely have limited my creativity.

For me, the Games programming exists in so many realms. It's an art, it's a test, it's theater, it's entertainment, it's community.

It's CrossFit.

*Sunday, April 9, 7:34 p.m.*
I haven't done much in the way of formal programming. When I say formal programming, I mean in my creative space, which I call Yarrow,

with my tools at hand. The tools are plenty of pads of paper and pencils, a whiteboard and dry erase markers, and the competition floor schematics I constantly have created and altered.

I've been doing what I normally do at this stage—even if I haven't been in my creative space. This means I'm giving the Games a lot of thought. Every moment I'm awake.

We are currently planning a trip to Madison in a few weeks to solidify a run-swim-run course. I'll dig into this more later, but for now understand this event is one of my staples for this year. I always have an event or collection of events that are going to set the tone for the entire weekend. These are my staples, or anchors.

Last year's major staple was the repeat of the Hero WODs Murph and DT from the 2015 Games. But they were not identical versions—they were slightly altered for 2016.

Another anchor in 2016: the return of the pegboard. I thought for sure the athletes were going to crush it the second time around. They didn't, and I was surprised.

In 2017, the anchor will be water events. I am planning on having the individuals and teams do two water events for the first time in CrossFit Games history. It was only six years ago that we introduced the water to the individuals and a couple of years ago that we introduced it to the teams.

Other knowns at this point include an obstacle course—a sprint version similar to the one we used at Camp Pendleton in 2012.

I am also going to bring back some heavy tests in weightlifting. I am thinking about having two heavy sessions. One day we'll test the Olympic snatch for one rep. On a second day we'll test a 1-rep-max clean and jerk. Or vice versa. These are great tests that play well to the crowd, and because we didn't do any barbell events in the Regionals, bringing them back to the Games in a big way sits well with me.

It's also time to put the speed ladders to bed for a year or two. I enjoyed those when we did them, and I like the way they played out, but I want to highlight raw strength isolated from strength while breathing hard.

Another idea floating around in my mind at this point is "*chaos.*" It's a developing idea I'll come back to.

Amanda is another benchmark CrossFit workout I am thinking about bringing back. Amanda was the first event on the schedule of the 2010 Games, the year we moved from The Ranch to the new venue in Carson *(named the Home Depot Center at the time)*. The Ranch is in Aromas, California, on the border of Monterey County and San Benito County. We were forced to scramble to find a new venue when Monterey County said events were not permitted on our agricultural land.

With the move to Wisconsin, it might be cool to bring Amanda back and make it the first event of 2017. Maybe not technically the first event, but the first event in the stadium. As of right now, the first events in Madison will be the water events—the run-swim-run. That said, at this stage we're early enough in the process that anything can be changed instantly.

*Saturday, April 15, 2:30 p.m.*
Yesterday, we finished up the Regional Director and Head Judge meeting. The purpose of the meeting was to go over the plan for Regionals. The CrossFit Games Regionals are the second phase of the season. To give you some perspective on how difficult it is to qualify for Regionals, we had 387,745 people from around the world compete in the first phase, the Open, which took place in winter. The best in the world meet in eight Regionals *(six in the U.S. and two overseas)*. This has been the format for the past few years. However, the Regionals were in an evolving state before then and will likely change again. The 2017 Regionals start in a few weeks.

The purpose of yesterday's meeting was primarily to introduce the Regional programming to the Head Judges and Regional Directors, all of whom attended this meeting. The teams talk in depth on logistical stuff surrounding the event, and representatives from Rogue Fitness—the equipment supplier for the Games—also attend this meeting. The gear is a big part of putting this all together.

These meetings are the first time most in attendance are told what the Regional events are. People can speak up and ask questions and point out potential problems. It's an invaluable process. I've often made changes based on these discussions.

Here's what happened this time: After I presented the slate of events to the group, we talked it through. Changes were made. I had an Individual workout that included wall balls with a 20-lb. ball, and the judges pointed out what they felt was a disparity between the Team and Individual categories. They thought that if we are making the teams use a 30-lb. medicine ball, we should make the Individual athletes use the 30-pounder, too. At first I resisted. But the truth of the matter is that their point was spot on. They were right. So we switched that Individual event to include a 30-lb. ball.

The thing about making this kind of change is that it can have a ripple effect. The med-ball change makes me worried about whether athletes will be able to complete the event under the time cap. I don't know because I haven't had the altered version tested. So that's precisely what I have to do.

I sent an email to James Hobart, who won the 2016 Central Regional as part of CrossFit Mayhem Freedom, and he's flying in Sunday night. I will have him test out the modified version Monday morning. I will probably also have him test the heavy deadlift workout, too. I can usually get a good read on a new or modified workout from my local testing athlete of choice, Matt Lodin. But I need someone at James' level to test the med-ball workout, especially if I have him available. Matt is a CrossFit Seminar Staff member and a great competitor. He has made it to the Regionals multiple years as an individual and on a team, and he's a great person to have locally for my tests. Last year he helped me test some Games workouts, and he even gave Dan Bailey (who finished fourth overall in the CrossFit Games in 2015) a run for his money on some of the events in the testing phase. He is also very knowledgeable about CrossFit programming and all things CrossFit, so his insight is invaluable.

We did the meeting at my private testing facility/creative space, Yarrow. Yarrow is the street the facility is located on, a few miles from my house. I have had it for several years now, and it has been crucial for my planning and process. I do a lot of the day-to-day CrossFit work at my home office, but when it's time to program or test workouts I come to Yarrow. It's where I can go to disconnect from everything else and focus with creativity. Using the two spaces has had an incredible effect for me. I recently learned that I function best when I have separate spaces for day-to-day work and big projects that are my responsibility.

Yarrow is about 3,500 square feet. Most of this is gym space. It has two Regional lanes set up with a Monster Rogue Rig structured with 11-gauge steel uprights. The construct is a simulation of the main-stage setup we use at the CrossFit Games. We have our floor lined with the same markings we use at our events. The perimeter of the space is lined with gear, basically all the gear we would ever use or have used at the Games. If you walk in from the outside and look around, it strikes you as a completely decked-out CrossFit affiliate.

We also have a few office rooms in the building. I use these as primary creative spaces to whiteboard the Games. I spend most of my time programming in these rooms. When I have a plan completely sketched out on the whiteboard, I can just walk out to the main gym floor and start setting up gear to physically see how the spacing of equipment works or doesn't work. Everything I need to test the ideas is at hand. It's an ideal lab for building a functional vision for the CrossFit Games.

During the Regional Directors meeting, I organized an epic knockout tournament. We have two basketball hoops in the indoor space. One is a portable hoop. The second is a hoop I rescued from a neighbor of mine who was throwing it out.

I learned how to play knockout a couple of years ago. It can be played with three people up to as many as you want. We even played it at the 2016 Games in one of our longer breaks.

During the meeting we had a tournament: five different rounds. Each was scored with the CrossFit Games scoring system. First place gets 100 points, second gets 94, and third gets 88. After that, points decrease by four per rank all the way down to 10th. Then it's down by 2 points to 40th place.

I finished ninth out of 21. I wasn't happy about that, but oh well. It's not the first time I wasn't happy with my performance. It won't be the last.

As usual, Head Judge Adrian Bozman was great. He has the ugliest shot you've ever seen, but it's a high-percentage shot. That and he just out-hustles everyone else on the floor. The winner of the overall tournament was Justin Bergh. His shot was on, and being 6 foot 5 he owned the boards and took home a nice cash prize. Anyone who wanted to play put in $20, winner take all. We had about 25 people play.

Bozman first got involved with CrossFit HQ teaching our Level 1 seminars a decade ago—his most important and consistent role with the organization. He technically weighs about 165 lb., but I like to say he presents like he is 185. Given his current combination of a mullet and curled handlebar mustache, Boz is a blend of biker gang and clean-cut hipster. Adrian is integral to the Games team as the Head Judge and a reliable person for me to bounce ideas off.

Justin Bergh is my second-in-command of the CrossFit Games. Where Adrian is shorter and stouter, Justin is tall and proper looking. He brings the professionalism to the team, and he has an *"industry look"* that differs from so many of us on the team or on CrossFit HQ staff. He brings a traditional sports background to the team but is without a doubt one of us—a true CrossFitter. He ran an affiliate, CrossFit Southside, before getting involved with the Games in 2009. He was also a member of our Level 1 Seminar Staff. Most of the head judges come from this group, and in 2009 he was on the judging team.

In the years after that, his role expanded and became more formal as the Games grew and he proved to be more valuable. When Tony Budding left a few years back, Justin's role as second-in-command—Games GM, we call him—became set in stone. Justin runs most of the day-to-day operations of the Games at this point. He manages hundreds of small moving pieces while I focus on the big picture and programming. We talk on a regular basis about the future of the Games, and we're in constant communication about all aspects of the competition season.

Finishing this meeting was key for me. Now that it's done, I can really focus on the Games and dive into the details and creation of the programming and schedule.

But after programming 10 other CrossFit Games, it doesn't come easy. It's sometimes hard to fire up the discipline I need to be creative, and it's hard to give it the attention it needs every day. Often I just find myself walking away from it for days on end. Honestly, I am doing that right now. But I will dive in and really start the creative process for the 2017 Games, most likely this evening or tomorrow.

*April 15, evening*

I did not dive back in like I had hoped. Instead I chose to take my two daughters, Zoë and Finley, to the beach. I am making this entry on my iPhone. It's not as easy to type on, but it works in a pinch.

Those who know me, people I consider friends and people I work with, know I have a family—a wife and two kids. Those who don't know me have no clue. I keep it that way by design. I have deliberately chosen to be very private with my family life and not put it out there for public consumption. You will never see me post anything about my family on social media.

I don't want my children to be recognizable to a bunch of strangers. Not only do I feel like it's more information than people need, but I also feel it's fundamentally not a safe practice. I know some CrossFit athletes and CrossFit *"celebrities"* who post so many pictures of their children that I could recognize their kids if I saw them on the street without their parents. I don't want that for my children or family.

I don't even feel comfortable with the frequency that I am recognized. It was never my goal or choice to be such a public figure in the CrossFit community. As my various roles in CrossFit evolved and the community expanded, it just ended up that way. I have become popular in this community, and it happens to be a really large community, so I get recognized a lot. I have decided not to force that on my wife or children.

I recognize that I am a very polarizing figure in CrossFit. Some people like me. Probably an equal number or more don't like me. Of all the people on social media that follow me, probably 99.9 percent are strangers. I have no interest in showing my family to these people or giving them that access. Not only do I have no interest, but I also have no reason. I don't owe it to anyone.

From my days in the Navy, I learned how to protect things, to compartmentalize and be what we called a *"silent professional."* It's been easy for me to keep my family out of the public eye. It's actually something I am very proud of, and I will continue to do it for my sanity, for their protection and for our future. It is by no means a reflection of how much I love them or care about them. I love my wife and children tremendously. When I have time off, I enjoy nothing more than just hanging out with them. We go on big trips from time to time, but I prefer family time at home these days after spending the last two decades in professions that have me traveling on a regular basis.

While I'm at the beach writing this, Zoë walks up and asks if *"Iceland Annie"* is going to go to the Games. Iceland Annie is Annie Thorisdottir, a two-time Games champion. I said she still has to qualify through the Regionals. Zoë replied, *"Please give her a VIP pass and just let her go. You can do that."*

*Monday, April 17*

Today we tested three Regional workouts with James Hobart. I had him fly in just for this purpose. He is not doing Regionals this year and is a perfect candidate to test events. In the CrossFit Open, he finished 33rd in the world, identifying him as one of the top CrossFit athletes around. It's great to have him available to test if needed. I don't use someone who is going to the Games to test an event that's going to be on the slate for the Games. That would obviously be highly unethical. Same with Regionals. If an athlete is going to compete in the Regionals, I won't ask him or her to test a Regionals workout. As for the Open, I never have a top athlete test a workout planned for the first phase of qualification.

We had an important event to test today:

CROSSFIT GAMES REGIONAL EVENT 3

FOR TIME:

100 DUMBBELL OVERHEAD WALKING LUNGES

100 DOUBLE-UNDERS

50 WALL-BALL SHOTS

10 15-FT. ROPE CLIMBS

50 WALL-BALL SHOTS

100 DOUBLE-UNDERS

100 DUMBBELL OVERHEAD WALKING LUNGES

TIME CAP: 16 MINUTES

At the Regional Directors meeting we raised the weight on the wall ball to 30 lb. from 20 and kept the reps at 50. Athletes do the sets of 50 twice. This is the first time we have included a 30-lb. wall ball in Regionals. As tested with Matt and a 20-pounder, it was completed just under the cap of 16 minutes. Because we made the change to 30 lb., I had to verify the workout would be appropriate for the Regional athletes with the same cap. At this stage of the process, the timing of the schedule is fixed. It can't change. If any components of the test change, I need to make sure I create something that fits in this 16-minute window.

James crushed it. He finished in 14 minutes and something, a good 2 minutes under the time cap. I was worried that nobody would be able to finish it, but James proved it's fine. I don't expect all athletes to finish, but that's OK. At the Regionals I am not programming for everyone. I am programming for the best.

We are still working out the height and weight of the wall ball for the women on this one.

I also had James test Event 4.

2017 CROSSFIT GAMES REGIONAL EVENT 4

FOR TIME:

60-FT. HANDSTAND WALK

10 TOES-TO-BARS

10 DOUBLE KETTLEBELL DEADLIFTS

60-FT. HANDSTAND WALK

12 TOES-TO-BARS

12 DOUBLE KETTLEBELL DEADLIFTS

60-FT. HANDSTAND WALK

14 TOES-TO-BARS

14 DOUBLE KETTLEBELL DEADLIFTS

60-FT. HANDSTAND WALK

16 TOES-TO-BARS

16 DOUBLE KETTLEBELL DEADLIFTS

The purpose of having him test this one was to verify the reps and weight on the kettlebell deadlifts, and his results confirmed that they are appropriate. He fought hard on the deadlifts, and that's what I wanted to see. He even broke up the toes-to-bars. He really enjoyed this one and thought it was grippy. The visual, how they look after testing something, is very important to me. I learn a lot about the test from those moments right after an athlete completes it. Did I get the result and stimulus that I wanted?

We had some time left, so we decided to have him test the final. The final isn't really too technical. It's just gassy. You need to move and move fast.

2017 CROSSFIT GAMES REGIONAL EVENT 6

FOR TIME:

30/25-CAL. BIKE

20 BURPEE BOX JUMP-OVERS

10 SANDBAG CLEANS

MEN USE A 30-IN. BOX AND A 150-LB. BAG

WOMEN USE A 24-IN. BOX AND A 100-LB. BAG

TIME CAP: 6 MINUTES

Jason MacDonald, one of our Seminar Staff members, a head judge and an ex-UFC star, actually did this one a few days ago at the Regional Directors meeting. His time ended up being faster than James': 4:17 versus 4:36.

After the three testing sessions we went to Five Guys for lunch, and James expressed that he wasn't happy about not beating Jason's time. But considering it was his third event in the span of a few hours, his performance was very impressive.

Now I feel that the tests are set, and I am going to erase the Regionals workouts from my wall and focus on the Games. It's the closing of one chapter in this season and the opening of a second.

After James left to head to the airport, I went back to Yarrow alone and cleaned up the walls in my space, erasing the Regional events. I spent some time looking at the Games schedule and figuring out where some things are going to go.

I am looking at doing Amanda for the Individual athletes, and that led me to consider doing Team Amanda. I started to play with what that would look like. Relay style with one continuous clock or six different scored events, like we did with the pegboard workout last year? Amanda, if it happens, will be on Thursday, the first workout we do in the Coliseum. I have committed to a Thursday-Sunday schedule for the Games. This will be the first time we do four days of continuous action and events.

I also just plugged in the snatch on Friday for individuals, and then the clean and jerk on Saturday. At this stage it's plug and play. Anything can move as it comes together.

I need to figure out what I will do for teams in terms of a heavy barbell test. They will get something in that realm for sure. I'm just not sure what yet.

Overall, I am very happy with the progress I made today. I cleaned my space and organized some things, and this is very important in my process for moving on to the next phase. Although this is not Day 1 of Games programming, it very much feels that way. I even had some ideas for 2019 that I am thinking through, but considering I want to release this book before those Games, I can't go too much into the details.

I have been following the CrossFit.com workout of the day for the past week or so. Today's workout was 30 rope climbs for time. I was worried about that because recently I have been getting overuse injuries in my arms from pulling. But I took it nice and slow—so slow that James made a couple of loving comments about my lackluster performance. So far I feel good doing the CrossFit.com WOD, but tomorrow's workout is going to eat me up.

*Tuesday, April 18, 9:35 a.m.*
Today's CrossFit.com workout was hard: 15-12-9 reps of 135-lb. thrusters alternating with 21-15-9 reps of 135-lb. sumo deadlift high pulls. That load is heavy for me in both movements. I remember a workout in 2008 or 2009 that had 135-lb. thrusters, and I was able to do a hard set of 12. Today I did 6 on the first set. I need to regain some strength and gas. Sticking to CrossFit.com will help with that.

As I was making the short drive from my house to Yarrow, today's workout caused a thought to pop into my mind. A lot of my ideas happen like this at random times. Today's idea: 21-15-9 reps of 135-lb. thrusters and burpees. Sure, we've done similar workouts in the Open, but it's different enough, and given the strength and speed of the top Games athletes, it would make for an epic test. Not much to do with this idea yet, but I will add it to the board as a potential sprint-type workout. I have a section of my whiteboard where I put ideas and things I might want to do. Often, these ideas move over to the actual working area, which means they end up in an event. Other times they stay where they are and never get used.

*5:01 p.m.*

I spent a few hours going over the schedule—one of the most time-consuming and difficult aspects of planning the Games. The schedule is everything. How long will the event take? How much time to get the athletes off the field? How much time to switch between events? There are a million things to take into consideration with the schedule, and I spend a lot of time on it. Sometimes events are made and the schedule is adjusted to accommodate them. Other times the schedule is made and events have to fit into it. I do almost all the scheduling work on a laptop connected to two other screens, giving me three in total. This year, because we have all divisions competing at the same time, we have a macro schedule, which shows all the events happening together on the same day, and a micro schedule, which details the Team and Individual competition schedules to the minute.

Today went well. I feel like I am getting back into the groove I had in summer 2016. Last year was the best year for programming the Games, largely because of this dedicated creative space. I'm able to leave the house and my home office and just come here to be creative or to sew—but we'll get to the sewing in another discussion.

I filled in some of the events for teams and individuals. I am going to place all of those, and then we can fill in the age groups.

I figured out the timing for the O-course: We will run it similar to 2012, using heats with eliminations. And I also gave some initial thought to how to run the teams through the O-course. Right now the idea is to do it relay style, but that will probably change.

I also broke out some paper and my pencils to figure out another event for the north lot: a *"work"* event, like a yoke carry with a flip and maybe a pull. We often do stuff like that, but the workouts are usually quick or paired with other things. I want to do one that is longer and just grunt work—farm work, because we will be in the Midwest. It will be fun to see where I take that one.

Something else I did today: toss the cyclocross event to John McLaughlin, aka Johnny Mac, aka J-Mac. Johnny Mac is one of the senior guys on our team. He runs all the Regional Directors and is great at logistics organization and leadership. He is truly an all-star on the team. I wish we had him in California, but he is a full-time firefighter in the Jupiter, Florida, area, so that job keeps him tied to the East Coast.

I asked him to plan the event out and present it to me so I can review and tweak it. Over the years, I have delegated parts of the Games to other members of our team, specifically the Masters competition. This might be the first Individual event I've delegated. But it's time for that. It's the right move, and it will allow me to focus on other aspects that need attention. Johnny is an avid cycler, and he understands my big-picture vision for the event. Plus, his work is always top notch and on time.

I'm going to leave Yarrow now. I'll be back tomorrow for another full session.

*Wednesday, April 19, 6:22 a.m.*
At 5:50, I was lying in bed thinking about the snatch and clean-and-jerk events. I thought, maybe we should repeat the overhead squat as a test instead of the snatch. It was a great event when we last did it, and I would like to see a handful of male athletes lift 400 lb. When I go to Yarrow today, I'll write this on the wall as a possibility.

*4:15 p.m.*
Just got to Yarrow. I made a little speed-bag video for an Instagram story to make fun of Dan Bailey. Now I'm diving into this year's actual schedule and template, plugging in events and playing with timing.

The schedule, logistics and flow of the Games are critical. We stay on schedule and we don't miss a timeline. But for that to happen, we have to design a schedule with execution in mind. Too often people make unrealistic schedules—or even life plans—they can't maintain, and then they fall off. So the schedule, while not sexy, is one of the things I spend most of my time on. And right now, I'm just working on this year's template (*while listening to Nirvana and The Doors*).

I made some good progress on a heavy lifting event for the teams. It will probably be a snatch, and I'm thinking of testing one gender on one day and the other gender the next day, so only three athletes from each team will lift at a time.

The challenge of heavy tests for the teams is coming up with a format that works in terms of logistics and isn't completely boring. They will do this event on the Coliseum floor, and I have a template to get them through quickly: Five lifters in the back row of platforms lift at once, and then the other five in the front row. We would get through three lifts by one athlete from each of the 10 teams in the heat in 3 minutes. Repeat that three times and we'll get every lifter on every team in the heat through three lifts in about 10 minutes.

Yesterday I also played with the idea of making the individuals do the run-swim-run on Sunday. Every year, the water event, and typically the longer events, are out of the way early in the Games. The run-swim-run won't be a super-long endurance event, but it is an endurance test nonetheless, and it is low impact enough that putting it on Sunday is very intriguing to me. I'll place it there for now.

Finishing up for the day, I was feeling good about where everything is. I made good progress with formatting the schedule, but once I started to dig in and really place things out, I am suddenly not feeling so great about it. I'm going to step away and take a break from everything. Time to reset.

I'm traveling up to Scotts Valley tomorrow for a meeting with Mercedes-Benz, which will force me to break from the programming routine and process that I am just settling into, but I'll continue to think about all this and come up with ideas.

*Thursday, April 20, 4:27 a.m.*

I woke up this morning thinking about pistols—not the kind you shoot but the single-leg squats that have been included in the Regionals but not the Open. I decided the athletes will see pistols in a big way at the Games. I don't know how yet, but it will be good.

*4:08 p.m.*

Just boarding an Alaska Airlines flight from San Jose back to San Diego. We had a good meeting with Mercedes-Benz and our team. They seem very interested in supporting the Games with some vans and maybe down the road doing a deal for our affiliates on Sprinter vans. I'm interested in seeing how this develops.

James was at the office for some other projects, so I was scheduled to have him test a workout with me at noon. But an hour earlier Sevan said Greg wanted to do lunch at Cafe Cruz. CrossFit Founder Greg Glassman and I are very busy, but in different ways, so I don't see him as often these days. I take the offer to hang with him any chance I get. Sevan Matossian is CrossFit's Director of Media. He and I couldn't have been more opposite when we met nine or 10 years ago. He is from Berkeley, and I was the hardcore MIL guy. He is a free spirit and hippie-like, and I am not really like that in the traditional sense. And so on. But we instantly hit it off and have been close friends since.

Back to James. I texted him to cancel the session and then quickly decided I can just get someone else to run it for me. CrossFit Games staff member Wilson Tang already knows the workout, so I tasked him with it. He and James met at 12:15 while I went to lunch, and they tested Regional Event 5: 21-15-9 reps of ring muscle-ups and overhead squats with an 80-lb. dumbbell. I think Matt Lodin did this event in around 9 minutes. I wanted to see how fast someone like James could do it, and I wanted to know what he thought of the reps, the pairing, the stimulus, etc.

James did it in 7:40.

*"Nobody is ready for that,"* he said via text, and I'm happy with that response. When I got back to the office, we talked about the workout. He didn't think it was going to be that bad or gassy, but it was both, so I'm excited to see this one play out at Regionals.

I haven't spoken much about Regional programming since I started this writing project, and now is not the time, either. I think I might wait until I start traveling for the Regionals to dive into them. I will also recap this year's Open at some point.

Another interesting thing happened on the way to the airport. Rich Froning texted me two workouts:

18-14-10

Muscle Up

9-7-5

Squat snatch 225#

Did a pegboard one the other day you might like

15 pegboard

150' hs walk

15 rope climb

150' hs walk

15 pegboard

(You could sub a bike or row, something to get heart rate up)

8:57 on muscle up/snatch

17 something on peg/hsw

Those are his notes and suggestions. Rich sends me his times on workouts he creates every now and then, and I appreciate it. He will send me things he does or combos he likes. I don't think I ever use any of them, but he for sure influences me in terms of potential loading, for example. As you now know, I'm considering doing heavy Amanda as the first workout in the Coliseum in Madison. I was thinking 185-215 lb., but seeing Rich's time on his muscle-up/snatch workout, I wonder if I should go 225.

I will eventually end up having a really good athlete, maybe even James, test these different versions after Regionals and in the summer before committing to the final version.

In the past, Rich has tested Individual events for me once he went team. But I didn't use him last year and probably won't use him this year. The process has changed because I have my lab to test the events.

On that note, I have a strong opinion on workouts versus tests. You do workouts in your gym. You work out to train for the Open, the Regionals and the Games. But you don't do *"workouts"* at Regionals and the Games. The Open tests are not workouts either. If you are registered for the competition, they are tests or events. It's a pet peeve of mine when people call them workouts.

Our plane is boarded. I don't have internet on this flight, and I'm working on Apple Pages, so I was planning to stop this writing session. I don't know if Pages works offline. But we're still on the ground, so I'll continue to work.

I'm going to talk a minute about Nick Urankar and a post I was made aware of today. Nick made a post about having to pay a $200 registration fee for Regionals and complained about how we are taking more of their money. I don't even feel like mentioning that all major sports have registration fees, but I'm disappointed because I feel like we are a smaller community of people who all know each other—and Nick knows me personally. I know his post is not a jab at me, but it's hard not to feel that way when I am the one who created this sport. His post pissed me off, but he's young and immature. I hope I don't have to deal with more of him in the future.

*Friday, April 21, 10:36 a.m.*
Today I did the first event in the Masters Online Qualifier, not because I qualified but because I am following CrossFit.com. The Masters Qualifier workouts will be the next four CrossFit.com workouts of the day.

Event 1 was hard: 100 dumbbell snatches, 80-calorie row, 60 burpees over the bar and 40 muscle-ups for time, with a 20-minute time cap. I had done 41 burpees when I hit the cap.

This programming is first created by Pat Sherwood and Stephane Rochet. They create what is essentially a first draft of tests and then present it to me. I usually modify, sometimes heavily, sometimes not much. I don't modify because anything they do is wrong but because I have a broader view of the season's tests.

For example, Pat submitted this year's programming for the Masters Online Qualifier with a 1-rep-max test. Because I decided the Regional programming wasn't going to have a 1RM test, I wanted to carry that theme and be consistent. Another big change was the first movement in Event 1. I think it was originally a barbell snatch. We changed it to 100 dumbbell snatches. The dumbbell was such a big implement in the Open—I really liked how that played out—and 17.1 ended with 50 dumbbell snatches followed by 15 burpee box jump-overs. So I thought it would be a nice continuation—and shitty—to see the first Masters event start with 100 snatches.

I've probably known Pat longer than anybody else in my life other than close family. I met him in 1998 when we were both in BUD/S (*Basic Underwater Demolition/SEAL training*). He was an officer and I was an enlisted guy. We ended up going to SEAL Team 4 together and became close friends. We stayed close for a number of years until our paths in the Teams took separate routes. We eventually reconnected when I was already working for CrossFit and offered him a job. He took the challenge and his been with us ever since.

Stephane Rochet is an ex-cop, ex-strength-and-conditioning coach for the University of San Diego and just all-around good guy. He stands 6 foot 5, and he's someone you don't want to run into in a dark alley, yet he scored 1590 on his SATs. His dad is a rocket scientist, and his brother scored a perfect 1600 on his SATs. Stephane works closely with me to oversee all the workout testing and floor design. He is a great member of our team.

*11:37 a.m.*
Spending more time on the schedule, making templates for the age-group divisions. Not really thinking about workouts today, just the logistics of the schedule.

*Saturday, April 22, 1:36 p.m.*
About an hour ago Jan-Willem Driessen, our main point of contact from 5.11 Tactical, texted to ask if we're planning on using vests at the Games this year. I've already made up my mind that we are not going to for the individuals and teams, but I suggested we might use them for the age groups. He said we could if we wanted to, so I've been thinking about this for the past hour—and I am thinking maybe we will use them again for the teams, too. I probably have to give them an answer sooner rather than later because they would have to make all those vests.

I also plan on using the litter again for the teams—I don't know how or where, but a litter event would be a good one for the team members to wear the vests. OK, this is playing out. I'm going to text him and ask if they can outfit the teams with vests.

It's a Saturday, not doing much yet. Might go to Yarrow and put in a real session. I leave in a few days for Madison, so I'll have a lot to see and decisions to make—namely on the run-swim-run.

*Sunday, April 23, 11:56 a.m.*

I did Age Group Online Qualifier #3 today. I scaled it because I am beat up from the previous two workouts and because I needed something a little faster with higher intensity. The workout is 21-15-9 reps of 135-lb. push presses and chest-to-bar pull-ups. I can do that, but it probably would have taken me 10 minutes or more. I scaled it to 105-lb. push presses and regular pull-ups, and it took me 4:17. That's exactly what I needed. Then I went for a little jog.

I like to run, and usually when I run I think about the Games or other work-related projects. Running helps me keep my mind active, and I get a lot of ideas in that mode. Today I was thinking about the experience and the schedule we are creating. In this whole process I have been thinking about ending the Masters competition at 3 or 4 p.m. with our new format. We can easily do that. But while running I thought, *"Why not spread their events out and let them end later in the day? Not exactly at 9 like the individuals will, but maybe at 6 or 7."*

Doing that will accomplish two things for the schedule and the event. First, it will give some breathing room throughout the day and limit the number of events going on at once. Second, it will give the people who just have Festival tickets a fuller day of competition to watch and enjoy. Both are very big positives, so I think we'll go in this direction.

I am watching MotoGP from Austin and Game 4 of the Cavs series. Once this is over, I will probably go to Yarrow and do some serious work.

*Monday, April 24, 10:04 a.m.*

I didn't make it to Yarrow yesterday to work on the programming, but I did come over to work on a project I am sewing for Greg. That took about two hours, added to the few other hours I put in on the same project last week. I came into Yarrow today and spent a little time finishing it off. Now I'm going to dive into some Games work.

Games work is what I'm best known for in CrossFit. I have been running this event for 11 years now. But I don't even consider that my most important role in CrossFit. My primary job in CrossFit is Director of Training. I co-direct that department with Nicole Carroll. We manage the training and education side of CrossFit and have been doing so for about 11 or 12 years. We oversee and manage all the seminars we conduct—Level 1, Level 2, CrossFit Kids,

Specialty Courses, etc., to include online courses. We have an international staff of over 175 trainers. They are the best in the world, and they travel globally to teach our methods to those who wish to be trainers or those who want to know more about CrossFit or a particular speciality in CrossFit.

This role takes up a significant amount of my time throughout the year even while I am working on the Games. But I will purposely not address that part of my job in this book. That part of my job—the lessons I have learned, the things we have accomplished—could be a book in and of itself. This book focuses only on programming and creating the CrossFit Games.

*10:53 a.m.*

I am not making much progress right now. I even feel slightly over-whelmed with it all, especially the schedule. I have finished all the templates I need for all the age groups. The templates I create are simply visuals and numbers I will plug into the schedule to show how long an event will take. For example, if I want to do a 15-minute heat, how long is it going to take all the divisions to get through on the master schedule? I made templates for all time possibilities and heat sizes. Currently, I'm working with 10 to 20 people per heat. We have a lot of divisions in the age groups (*14-15, 16-17, 35-39, 40-44, 45-49, 50-54, 55-59, 60+*), and because other divisions are competing at the same time, it's important to know how long any group can be on a floor before having to move for the teams or individuals.

I am starting to have my doubts now. This happens often in the process of programming, and when it does it really sucks, but I will come around. I usually handle these situations in one of two ways: I completely step away or I push through. Right now I plan on using the step-away technique to deal with it.

*Tuesday, April 25, 8:31 a.m.*

I am currently on a flight to Denver, with a final destination of Madison. My goal for this trip is to figure out the run-swim-run course and see if it will work as I envision it. The event will be a major part of the Games this year because all divisions will do it. I also want to open it up as a spectator event, too—fans can do the same course every Games athlete does.

This part of the process is important for me: actually seeing, and in this case running, the course. I am very visual with these events. I can't commit to an event without seeing it or running the course first.

When the Games were in Carson, it was much easier. I would just drive the 1.5 hours to L.A. and verify the course or venue as needed. Now that the Games are halfway across the country, going to Madison is a full trip: an entire day out and an entire day back.

Including the Open announcement we did a few months ago, this will be my fifth trip to Madison since the whole process of moving the Games started.

Another goal I have for this trip is to visit a bunch of the local affiliates. I have a goal of visiting all the affiliates in the local area as soon as I can. I think there are 18 of them, and I have already visited two. Hopefully I can visit three to six on this trip. It will take a few more trips to get them all.

Back to the main reason for the trip: the run-swim-run. Here's how it came to be an event.

During the process of selecting a new city to host the Games, Justin, Billy Rodgers, Danny Rodgers and I toured the three most interested potential hosts: Jacksonville, Florida; Chattanooga, Tennessee; and Madison, Wisconsin. *(Danny and Billy are brothers who own Framework Events, a company we contract to run a lot of the Games logistics. The two have worked with us for a number of years and created this company basically to service the Games. They are great members of the team and provide tremendous value in the whole system.)*

All three cities were friendly and could easily host triathlons. A big plus for the cities of Chattanooga and Madison was that they had both hosted actual Ironman events. Our points of contact for the two cities raved about those events and used them as selling points as to why we should and could hold the Games in their cities. They also spoke very highly of the event organization and the type of athlete the Ironman brings to the city.

Frankly, I was sick and tired of hearing about Ironman triathlons by the end of the tour. I mentioned that as Justin and I were driving over the 17 from the San Jose airport to our Scotts Valley office. He told me he had read a book on Ironmans and how they were created. He said a Navy officer created the first Ironman to settle a debate about which athletes were the best. I hadn't heard that. Justin was really into the history and the fact that the Ironman had that storyline to it.

Separate from this, we had some interest and pressure from HQ colleagues who were advising us to get involved with an obstacle-course race or potentially do our own. Personally, I hate the idea of an obstacle-course race, but

I love the idea of a mass-participation event. Our Open is obviously that, but it's online, and none of our physical events allow mass participation.

A typical CrossFit event can't allow mass participation like a 5K, triathlon or obstacle-course race because CrossFit events need judges to maintain the standards and count reps. As long as I am involved, we will uphold these standards in any event that CrossFit HQ does. It's our job to do that.

But those other events can have hundreds and even thousands of participants because they are held on a set course and every individual doesn't need a judge.

To me, the obstacle-course thing was and is played out. It's a fad, which is funny for me to say because people say our sport, our methodology, is a fad. It's not something I want our brand or our sport to jump on because it's so popular right now. We could do a run as a mass-participation event, but that's being done, and the space is already saturated.

Back to Justin and his story about how a Navy officer created the Ironman Triathlon. He asked me what I thought about triathlons and if I did them when I was in the Navy. I said there were two camps of people: those who did them and those who hated them—and 90 percent of us hated them. Very few guys actually did or were into triathlons, but we all did run-swim-runs.

And that's when it hit me: Run-swim-runs were a common training tool and test for us in the Navy. They were easy to do in terms of selecting a course, and they could handle large numbers. You also didn't need any special gear such as an expensive bicycle.

At that moment, at the tail end of that discussion, it clicked for me. That's our mass-participation event: the run-swim-run. Nobody else is doing it currently. It's an original idea that has a great story to it, and it connects with my history and who I am in this community.

The fact that it is mostly new and original to the U.S. in an organized fashion makes me think it can be a hit. It can be a CrossFit-run mass-participation event that gets people out of their boxes, garage gyms and typical CrossFit routines to do something really cool and completely scalable.

Now to the Games. The Games, in my eyes, are going to be the test for this event and something that helps build a lot of interest if we decide to do a mass-participation event. I think it's a great idea. I don't know if we will ever pull it off, but I like the idea of trying to scale the event. But we have to focus on our priorities, and at this point, a mass-participation event is not a priority for CrossFit.

I will see and run the course tomorrow, minus the swim. Then I will see how many people can fit on it at once. That's an important factor. Can 50, 100, 500 run it at once?

I would like to run the Individual men and women, 80 athletes, as one heat all at the same time. I am a big fan of having them compete at the same time in identical efforts so you can see female athletes beat men. I love that—like when Sam Briggs beat 90 percent of the male field in a run through the hills of my family's ranch last year at the Games.

I'm thinking about putting this event on Sunday. We have never done a swim event or a typical endurance event on Sunday at the Games. Typically, Sunday features a few shorter workouts that lead into the finale. But putting this on Sunday would be a nice twist, and I am comfortable with it because this event will be longer but very low impact. It will also force athletes to push for longer at a stage when they are typically worn down and tired. And I like that angle, testing mental toughness when the comp is almost over.

I would like to do a complete six-person relay for the teams on this event: One person does the complete course and tags the next person. Repeat a total of six times. I understand this could take a very long time, but I'm willing to consider it at this stage.

For the age groups, we have them broken into three smaller groups: 35-39/40-44/45-49 (120 athletes), 50-54/55-59/60+ (120 athletes), and 14-15/16-17 (80 athletes). I would like each group to able to start and finish all together. Depending on the size of the course, that might be hard to accomplish. When I speak of size, I mean the width of the run route specifically. In the water, the numbers are not an issue to me because the athletes will be spread out by the time they get there.

The course I am planning is around 1.5 miles long on the first leg. I haven't decided on the swim, but somewhere between 500 and 750 yards. I think 1,000 will be too long, especially for inexperienced swimmers. And then about 1.5 miles on the final leg.

As I said earlier, the individuals will go on Sunday, but the other groups will go at different stages throughout the week. I'm thinking the teams will go on Thursday, and then the age groups will get plugged in at various points on Friday and Saturday.

Something else that's exciting about this plan is the fact that this is the first time the age-group athletes will swim. I wonder if they're preparing for that test.

I'm excited about seeing this course and what's possible. I really want it to work, and I would like to try to scale this to make it our mass-participation event. I want to own the run-swim-run space. When people who are not SEALs hear that term, I want them to think of CrossFit.

One final thought: This past winter, Justin went out to Wodapalooza to check out their event. I don't follow those events or their workouts, so I have no idea what they do. I deliberately don't watch them or look at their programming. When Justin texted me and said, *"You will never believe this, they did a run-swim-run as one of their events,"* my initial reaction was, *"Ah, fuck. That sucks."* But it also doesn't discourage me from wanting to do our event. I imagine people will say we copied them, but with my history in these events, I hope not. Justin also said that the original Wodapalooza event was to be a run-paddle-run, but the winds were too high for the paddle so they changed it to a swim. So at least it wasn't their original planned event. They also did the run on a TrueForm Runner.

*Wednesday, April 26, 1:52 p.m.*
Yesterday evening I arrived in Madison at around 4 p.m. and started off with my box drop-ins right from the airport. We've hosted a few dinners for the local affiliates during our other trips here, and during those dinners I've mentioned that I will visit each and every box. When I say something like that, it is very important to me to honor my word and follow through. So part of this trip involves visiting as many of the affiliates as I can.

Yesterday evening I was able to see four. This morning I woke up at 6 and was able to visit another four. One was closed. This afternoon I will try to visit another two or three.

But the main purpose of my trip is to test the running portions of the run-swim-run course. I met Danny at the facility around 10 a.m. The first thing I did was a 15-minute live stream to Instagram to talk about the venue and the upcoming Games. I started a Twitter account a few days ago, and I also posted some pictures from the venue to that account.

It was pouring rain, but I am on a tight timeline, so I wasn't going to let that prevent us from running the course. We ran and we got soaked.

The first leg of the run starts between the arena and the convention center. It essentially runs in front of the Coliseum and then makes a hard left to run down a nice large road for a good distance. The early part of the route will provide some room for people to spread out. The run will then go across a grass field to the left of the dog park and link up with an existing trail. The trail isn't incredibly large, but it will work for this event. You run down the trail, cross a bridge, go under two separate overpasses and end up at the water. It's a great route that never crosses any roads.

Once we got to the water we discussed some of the logistics of the event and how the water section would go down—how athletes will take off their shoes and how they would know which are theirs. They will all be issued essentially the same shoes by Reebok.

*(As I'm typing this and thinking about the logistics at the water, I had a great idea about how to start for the teams, so I quickly sent Danny a note.)*

Danny had a really good suggestion to have the athletes put their shoes on rubber mats with their names on them. We worked out some more of the details on that and then ran back via the same route.

On the run back, we found a way to use a different section to prevent cross traffic, and we discussed how this would go down.

I'm thinking the Individual male athletes will go, with the women maybe two or three minutes later. I would prefer all 80 go at once, but we will see.

For teams, a straight relay.

The largest group will be the age-group athletes, with up to 120 athletes in one section. The teenage group is much smaller at 80. We might have to start by division. After that, we walked the venue floor to discuss some aspects of the Coliseum, then went into the pavilions and discussed those areas.

Finally, we looked at the outdoor competition floor. Building it will be a huge expense, but we have to do it. We're in the early stages of working that out.

*8:56 p.m.*

Just got back to the hotel after a long, long day of visiting affiliates and driving all across Wisconsin. It was very rewarding and relaxing. I'm happy I did it—13 affiliates visited in about 30 hours.

Trusting my team and delegating roles have allowed the Games to grow so fast. I'm able to delegate to people I trust so I don't hold things up.

For example, Stephane, Adrian and Pat are in Columbus filming complete video standards for the Regional events. In the past, I would have insisted on being there. I would have needed to be there. Yesterday, Stephane texted me throughout the day to ask questions about some of the events and possible changes.

After my last affiliate visit, I was driving back to Madison on some back road, and I decided I should call Stephane and go over his questions. When I called, Stephane, Adrian and Pat were all in a room figuring out what they had left to do, so I was able to talk to the three of them on speakerphone.

One question they had was about making the Worm/rope-climb event 5 rounds instead of 6. Our demo team in Columbus did it with a light Worm, like 75 lb. versus 455, and barely finished under the cap. So the guys were concerned that teams might not finish. I actually pushed to keep it as is. I'm OK if a lot of teams don't finish because the top teams will. And they'll have to hustle to get it done—I hope. We'll see in a few weeks.

Another question was about the reps in another Team event. We dropped the chest-to-bar pull-ups from 150 to 125. I originally had that event tested at 100 but moved the number up to make it harder. Turns out 150 was too many to finish under the time cap. It was a good call. They are a good team, and I have all the confidence in the world in them. I'm lucky to have them on board.

*Thursday, April 27, 10:02 a.m.*

I'm on my flight home from Madison. On the flight out here, I finished a book from a Madison author about his motorcycle trips, and I started a book by Tiger Woods on winning the 1997 Masters. This is going to lead me to talk about three things: reading, Tiger Woods and my career as a SEAL.

At the end of 2015, Erik Preston, another solid member of our Seminar Staff and a Head Judge at Regionals and the Games, gave me a book to read. It was fiction: *"The Martian."* The book was eventually made into a very successful movie starring Matt Damon. I have been an avid reader throughout my life. As a kid I read a lot of books, mostly science fiction, Dungeons & Dragons types of books. I also read *"Jurassic Park"* and *"Rising Sun,"* both by Michael Crichton, and *"Shogun."* I remember reading that last one because it was so long.

I eventually switched to reading books about Bruce Lee and karate, another thing that really held my interest as a child. Once I became interested in something, I would consume all the available books on the topic.

Then I got into the military and SEALs, so I started reading all those books—all Dick Marcinko's books and any other book I could find on being a SEAL, SEAL training or anything related. That laid the foundation for me to stop reading fiction books.

I went into the Navy, and in that career I read a lot, but no fiction. I read mostly instructional guides for what I was into, and at that time I was mostly into climbing, so I read a lot of books on climbing—how-to books and testimonials, true stories of climbing adventures. I read, but not as much as I would like.

I believed that if I was going to spend time reading, I should read nonfiction and learn something from it. I believed there wasn't much to learn from fiction. That carried through most of my adult life, even through my early CrossFit years. My books of choice in the early stages of getting involved with CrossFit were obviously nutrition and fitness books. That continued all the way to December 2015, when Erik gave me *"The Martian."* It was a gift, so I decided I should give it a go: *"It's December, and I have some down time, so let's tackle it."*

*(Others have given me fiction books that I still have not read. Froning gave me a "Gates of Fire"-like book that still sits on the shelf. Maybe I will eventually get to that. I've also been gifted SEAL books that I won't read. More on that later.)*

So I picked up *"The Martian"* and started reading it. I was instantly captivated by the book. It was fun and stimulating, as good fiction is. I read the book in a couple of days. Once I start something and really enjoy it, I kind of go all in, so finishing a book I enjoy in a matter of days is usually not that hard for me.

As 2015 was coming to a close, I made a goal for myself for 2016. I wouldn't call it a new year's resolution because I think those are almost always easily abandoned or broken in a matter of months. I made a three-part goal:

1. Read more.

2. Read only fiction.

3. Read only classics or works considered books of significance.

This goal was easy to accomplish. I read over 25 books in 2016, most of them classics, including a handful of epic 1,000-page books, and I made a discovery: There is plenty to learn from fiction.

Some of those books included *"The Grapes of Wrath," "East of Eden,"* and *"Of Mice and Men,"* all by John Steinbeck, who is a favorite of mine because he grew up in and wrote about the area in which I grew up. I also read *"Les Misérables"* by Victor Hugo, *"The Odyssey"* by Homer, *"Atlas Shrugged"* and *"The Fountainhead"* by Ayn Rand, and *"The Sun Also Rises"* by Hemingway.

This goal will now be part of my routine and part of who I am for the rest of my life.

Years ago, I went to William Buckley's speaking school. One evening, the class went to his house for dinner. I will never forget that his living room and basically every wall in the house was cluttered with books—more books than I had ever seen in my life. I was blown away. It left a lasting impression on me. I asked him about it, and he said he reads every day multiple times throughout the day. I didn't know how it was possible. But now I understand. And now I see the importance of doing it.

Including reading as part of my standard routine has given me new life and energy. It keeps me fresh, keeps my mind stimulated and gives me some adventure to dive into every day. It takes my mind off distractions and things I should ignore. It has done wonders for keeping me off of social media, specifically Instagram. If I find myself spending too much time on Instagram, I simply put the phone down and pick up my book. I believe reading has helped me perform all my jobs, including programming the CrossFit Games, at a higher level.

This year, 2017, I have loosened up my 2016 goal. I'm still reading, but I've let nonfiction creep back in. I will also read books that are not classics. But when reading fiction, I bias to classics over modern books.

Which leads me to the book I am reading now: "*The 1997 Masters*" by Tiger Woods. I picked this book up because I have always been a huge fan of Tiger Woods, his athletic career and his story. Some of that has to do with the time I spent with him when I was a Navy SEAL.

Before I get to the Tiger Woods story, I have to address being a Navy SEAL.

I have always told myself that if I ever wrote a book, I would not mention the words "*Navy SEAL.*" I feel like I was raised in that community correctly, and I took to heart the message of being a silent professional. I truly believe that what we did, why we did it and how we did it should not be shared with the world or boasted about—either while performing the job or after leaving the military. A select group held or holds the job, and secrecy is of the utmost importance. I still feel strongly about that, even out of active duty for almost eight years.

But in writing this book, I have to talk about myself and the things that made me who I am. I realized it will be very hard for me not to mention being a SEAL. The fact of the matter is that it is such an important part of my life—who I am and what I did. What I can do, though, is minimize the amount I talk about it. This book, or any I write in the future, will not be known as a Navy SEAL book or a SEAL memoir even though the author was a SEAL. This is a book about the programming of the CrossFit Games and a peek into what that takes. It happens to be written by a former Navy SEAL.

When I first got involved with CrossFit HQ in about 2006-2007, I was still on active duty, and it was very important to me that I kept the Navy job out of the picture. I continually reminded Greg, and Tony, not to mention that I was a SEAL and not to post about it, and they were good about that. They understood I didn't want that out there. And for years it wasn't. Those closest to me knew I was a SEAL, but most in the community did not. Even now, not that many people know I was a SEAL. I still run into people who say, "*Dave, I had no idea you were a Navy SEAL until I listened to Julie's podcast or read such-and-such article.*"

The first time I started talking about it in interviews or on camera was in 2010, after I got out of the Navy. Even if you look at my social media now or how I present myself, you will see I do not lead with *"former SEAL."* I don't want to be defined that way. I never wanted to be Dave Castro the Navy SEAL. I needed to start fresh in this community and be defined for who I am here and what I do here.

A lot of guys have written books and a ton of movies have been made. Instagram account bios prominently feature *"Navy SEAL,"* and the accounts' pictures are nothing but photos that show how cool the owners once were. I have friends who have done this and continue to do it. I personally don't agree with this way of handling who we were and what we did, but I also understand that it's how some of them are trying to put food on their tables for their families or how they're trying to make something for themselves after leaving the Navy. I am fortunate enough that I didn't have to do that because I had a great job waiting when I left the Navy. I had the opportunity of a lifetime, and I was able to seamlessly leave the Navy and build my life around a career that had nothing to do with my previous occupation.

I am incredibly proud of what I did. If it wasn't for CrossFit, I would have stayed in the Navy for 20 years, and at this stage I would be getting ready for retirement. But I'm disappointed by those in our community who don't follow the silent-professional ethos that at one time was so defining of who we are and what we stand for. I will continue to be that person, and I will stay the silent professional. I won't share war stories publicly, and I won't share with the world what we did and why we did it.

Back to Tiger Woods. ESPN The Magazine recently published a story that talked about his working with the SEAL teams and other aspects of his life. The author who wrote the article had called and left me a voice message something like this: *"Dave Castro, I know that you were a SEAL Qualification Training instructor around these years, and those are the years that Tiger Woods trained there. Can I ask some questions for my article?"*

I was impressed that he had pieced it together, so I talked to him. Yes, I was an instructor when Tiger Woods would come out and shoot with us. He probably came out two or three times. He probably has no recollection of me, although we once had a conversation in which I tried to convince him to do Fran. We were driving down from our instructor barracks to the shooting range.

*"Tiger, I heard you are pretty fit. There is this workout I think you should give a try,"* I said.

*"What is it?"*

*"It's 21-15-9 thrusters and pull-ups."*

*"How much weight is on the bar, and what is a thruster?"*

I saw Tiger processing. I described the weight and the movement, and he was deep in thought. We got down to the range, and he was getting ready to take a photo with the class. He asked me for more information.

*"Describe the thruster to me again."*

After I described it again, he respectfully declined to do it. I think he made a mistake. He could have discovered CrossFit then, most likely had a healthier career and broken all the records he missed. Or at least that's how I will believe his future could have been with CrossFit.

The author of the article wanted to verify some stories he had heard about Tiger's time with us. This conversation was not one he knew about. I didn't volunteer it, either. I hadn't heard most of the stories he asked me about, and I said I could not verify them. And that was the truth. They were pretty off-the-wall stories. The one story I could verify was the time we all went to a small diner near our shooting range for lunch. It was a favorite of ours for a good bacon cheeseburger. About six of us, including Tiger, sat around a circular table. We had our burgers and told some stories. He sat mostly quiet, and then the waitress came up with the check and asked whom it should go to. The table became silent. We had hosted other people before from outside of our community. Adidas execs, NFL football players, even family members, and out of respect they always picked up the tab because of the access we had given them and what we allowed them to do.

After a long, awkward silence, our chief at the time said, *"Separate checks, please,"* and the lady brought over six different checks to a group that included Tiger Woods. Tiger didn't pick up the tab.

We were all baffled by that. I struggled with understanding it for a long time. I just think he is a very odd dude who never really knew a normal life, and obviously years later we found out he had a lot of things going on.

I verified that story as true and asked the author not to mention me in the article. I didn't want to be mentioned in an ESPN piece on Tiger Woods and perhaps get dragged into that whole mess.

To this day, I am still a fan of Tiger Woods, and I watch every golf tournament he tees up on. I would love to see him come back to the brilliance he once had and break the records for major victories and PGA tour victories. I still hold out hope and believe that he can.

Oh, and I'm almost done with his book. It was two easy reading days, both on flights, and I will be done by the time we land. I enjoyed it. Good book.

Heal up fast, Tiger, so you can come break some records. And I would love to take you to lunch. I'll pick up the tab.

*Friday, April 28, 9:01 a.m.*

I just posted a photo announcing the inclusion of the 5.11 weight vests for Regionals. I was looking at some of the activity around the post and came across something Lauren Fisher posted a few days ago. It's a post about her running on a TrueForm. Well, at least that's what I thought on first glance. I looked closer at the video and it turns out she's on an Assault AirRunner. In the text she thanked Assault for lending a runner for training. My anger level spiked instantly.

The AirRunner is a new piece of equipment we are going to use at Regionals. It's made by the company that makes the AirBike. Roger Bates, the owner, is a good friend of mine. I have used the AirRunner and the TrueForm. The AirRunner is very different from the TrueForm, which most athletes in our community have experience on.

The AirRunner doesn't get released for purchase until after Regionals, so no athlete had access to it or the ability to train on it before Regionals. That needed to be consistent. Nobody gets to use it prior to Regionals. I actually spoke at length with Roger about this before agreeing to use the AirRunner in Regionals, and he agreed not to let any athletes see it before the competition. Those who train on it would have a distinct advantage over those who couldn't. We discussed this, so Lauren's post pissed me off.

I sent Roger a text. He hasn't responded yet. I then sent him and Traci an email. *(Traci Bates is co-owner of Assault.)*

Things like this frustrate me so much. I try to maintain the integrity of the competition and what we do, but sometimes people don't think of the bigger picture and undermine the event by doing things like this.

The good news is that we have not announced the workouts yet, so someone like Lauren, who has access to the AirRunner early, won't be able to train for the exact event. Once Roger calls me back, I will probably tell him to pick the AirRunner up and take it back before the events are announced. Again, this is only a problem in that it's not available to every other athlete before Regionals. If it were, it would not be an issue. But it's not available.

Oh well. Moving on.

I'm currently working on plugging Masters time blocks into the Games schedule.

*Saturday, April 29, 7:05 p.m.*
Didn't do much programming today. I decided to go to the Level 1 Certificate Course at CrossFit Del Mar. I trained with the Seminar Staff at lunch. It was fun and humbling. I got crushed by all the staff members. Later, I had a sewing-machine repairman come fix one of my machines, which turned into getting two of them fixed.

*7:22 p.m.*
I did some more work plugging in the schedule blocks for the age groups. I'm getting excited, but I'm nervous. I'm starting to have some doubt that this whole plan is going to work. This is the first time the entire competition will happen over the course of four days. But I know it will execute beautifully because of our preparation. I just need to keep reminding myself of that.

*Sunday, April 30, 2:57 p.m.*
I spent a few quality hours on the schedule plugging and playing with where the Masters events will go. I have a meeting with Stephane and Pat here tomorrow, so I need to get an idea of what I expect Pat to do with regard to the Masters programming. In the previous two or three years, I let him and a team program and present me the workouts without regard for the Team and Individual events. In years past, the age groups competed before the teams and individuals. This year, everything is happening over four days. I'm going to have the masters do some of the same stuff the individuals do.

Like the run-swim-run, and the obstacle course, and possibly a version of the work/farm event I'm creating.

While plugging in these workout blocks, I was thinking of an event we could do in the dog park. Currently there is nothing in the dog park other than the bike course we are creating for the individuals.

So I started playing with the idea of a 400- or 800-meter run course. At this point, the only other running is in run-swim-run, but that's more of an endurance test than running in a classic CrossFit test. So it would be good to have a run between 400 and 800 meters in a CrossFit workout.

I don't really want to use the AirRunner at this stage, not because Roger fucked up and pissed me off the other day but because that style of running is for Regionals. When we host big events like this, we run outside. That's the beauty of the Games: It's a single event and doesn't have to be replicated like Regionals that are hosted over several weekends around the world. Back to Roger: He is a great guy with a huge heart. He cares about the community and has made some really cool equipment for it.

As I was thinking about the dog-park area and the run, I was thinking about what else we could do with it. A clean might be cool—maybe a clean with a med ball or uneven object just because there is not much flat land at the dog park. Because the ground is so uneven out there, barbell and rig work don't make much sense. I am thinking this event will be for the masters only, but there's a small chance we can make it an Individual or Team event, too.

One of the big things I will go over with Pat and Stephane: the number of events for each age group.

During 17.5 in Madison, we had a quick meeting with Justin, J-Mac and Stephane, and we agreed to something like this: For the three divisions in the 35-49 group, one workout on Thursday, three on Friday, three on Saturday and one on Sunday. For the three divisions in the 50-60+ group, one on Thursday, two on Friday, two on Saturday and one on Sunday. For the Teen divisions, we decided on the same number as the older Masters grouping. But as I was sitting here playing with the schedule and number of events, I decided to create a three-event day for the Teens on Sunday. They're young. They can handle it.

This will be the first time the masters compete for four days. So we have to give a lot of thought to load and volume. This will also be the first time the masters truly have different programming for different age groups. Some of the events will be the same, but some will be tailored to the age group, meaning we won't just program an event for the 35-39-year-olds and expect everyone else to do it, too. That's how we've done it, and it worked because CrossFit is infinitely scalable. But this year's programming will be so much better because of this new format.

I'm excited for a possible med-ball/run event. I also thought to add lifting a med ball over a wall, with the athlete jumping over, too. During this programming session, I emailed Bill Henniger and asked him to look into making some walls for the dog park.

Bill is the owner and founder of Rogue Fitness, the global gear behemoth that supplies equipment for a majority of our community and various others out there.

Bill wasn't always a huge player in the gear industry. I first met him at a CrossFit Level 1 Certificate Course I was teaching in 2006 or 2007 at CrossFit Ann Arbor in Michigan. It was late on Day 2, and I was heading out to catch a flight back home. Bill came out and asked if he could speak to me for a minute. He introduced himself and handed me some jump ropes and maybe some rings. He said he was starting a gear company and would love to be involved in helping at the Games. I told him to stay in contact, and I gave him my email address. He stayed in contact and then ended up helping at the 2009 Games, mainly with plyo boxes. After that his role grew every year, just as his company experienced exponential growth. Our working relationship and personal relationship grew, too. Bill is someone I can rely on to get the job done and get it done well. He has built a great team at Rogue, and it's largely because of his no-bullshit attitude and dedicated work ethic. Not many people work harder than Bill.

Over the years, when I have random and crazy ideas, I've sketched them out and sent them to Bill. *"Is this possible?"* I ask. Often he says *"no."* Then a few days later he comes back and says, *"I think it can work."* Almost every time, he ends up providing me with a prototype regardless of what he originally thought of the idea. This became a two-way street. After I fed him ideas for a few years, Bill started shooting me some ideas and proposing things Rogue could do. The back and forth has led to great events in Carson, and hopefully it will lead to great events in Madison—events with specialized gear the athletes have not seen before and aren't prepared for.

Oh yeah: Bill's wife Caity, formerly Caity Matter, is the 2008 CrossFit Games Champion.

Overall, I'm in a good programming head space, although I'm still not getting into the exact details of workouts/tests. That comes later. Figuring out this massive schedule is very important, and I have been chipping away here at Yarrow for about three hours.

Tomorrow's meeting with Pat and Stephane will be good.

## MAY 2017

*Monday, May 1, 3:43 p.m.*

I had a good meeting with Pat and Stephane. We talked about the event time blocks and the actual events I had plugged in for the Age Group athletes, and Pat was happy and excited about the things we are making them do. When I told Pat about the clean event with maybe burpees, he was very excited about that. He had tested something very similar on his own.

We didn't dive into specific workouts he had created at this point. I don't need those distractions. I gave him freedom to create those workouts, and we can go over them much later. What's most important at this stage is getting his timing down to match the schedule we are creating. Now he will take the blocks I created and look at actual timelines for some of the events.

After that, I went to the leather store to pick up some new leather to sew with. On the way out I got a text from a friend of mine, Grace Patenaude, owner of Atomic CrossFit in Stafford, Texas. She said there was some discussion and complaints that the masters did not have their own Regional event. Every year we hear that argument. The numbers have never really supported doing it—especially in the older divisions. In age groups where only a few hundred or a few thousand compete, why have Regionals?

As time has passed, and especially after this year, I really like the Online Qualifier as a second stage after the Open. I have some good ideas on how to make it better for next year, too. It's possible we'll have a workout or two that they must perform and submit on the same day it's announced, kind of like a *"virtual Regional."* We might also tie announcements to it. If we did announcements, I would not do them—maybe someone from the team. All these ideas still need to develop, and there will be time for that after the Games. For now, I need to focus on Games planning.

*Tuesday, May 2, 8:29 p.m.*

I am on a flight up to HQ for another meeting that isn't related to the Games. I will be there for the next three days, Tuesday to Thursday. I'll have some time to meet with Justin and the Games team and get some good planning in. When I meet up here with these guys, it's less about the programming and more about big-picture stuff and event stuff: the flow of the weekend, the spectator experience, the judges, the media and all of that. One million questions need answers.

Because I'm on a flight and have the time to write, I want to reflect on this year's Open. This is the story of the 2017 Games programming, so I might as well talk about the entire season. I will cover the Regional programming in depth, but it seems appropriate to do it once I start traveling for Regionals in a few weeks.

17.1

10 DUMBBELL SNATCHES

15 BURPEE BOX JUMP-OVERS

20 DUMBBELL SNATCHES

15 BURPEE BOX JUMP-OVERS

30 DUMBBELL SNATCHES

15 BURPEE BOX JUMP-OVERS

40 DUMBBELL SNATCHES

15 BURPEE BOX JUMP-OVERS

50 DUMBBELL SNATCHES

15 BURPEE BOX JUMP-OVERS

MEN USE 50-LB. DUMBBELL AND 24-IN. BOX

WOMEN USE 35-LB. DUMBBELL AND 20-IN. BOX

I was very pleased with how 17.1 turned out. I wanted to have a test that used dumbbells. It would be the first time we included them in the Open, and I wanted it to be a bruiser, something that hurt. I also wanted to kick off the Open with an event for time. For-time events, generally speaking, have more intensity and greater consequences than tests programmed for a certain amount of time. Cindy, Fight Gone Bad and most of the Open events we have done are performed for a set amount of time, so you know the clock will save you eventually. You can pace a little more. But if you have to complete a certain number of reps to stop the clock, pacing is still important but you really need to keep the pedal to the metal throughout to get a good time.

I tested different versions of 17.1—a version with fewer burpees overall, a version in which burpee and snatch reps increased, a version in which both the burpee and snatch reps were fixed. I tested earlier versions before I was happy with it, and I had Matt test it. I think I ended up having him test two different versions, and I was happy with how it played out.

For the actual 17.1 announcement, we decided to do the announcement from Paris, France, and the trip out went great. When I travel for the Open, especially internationally, I am usually in and out quickly. But for this trip I decided to come out early in the week, do the announcement, stay a day and then come home on Saturday.

On the way out, the travel actually hit me pretty hard. I didn't adjust quickly. But my schedule was rough to begin with. Our announcement was going to be at 2 a.m., so we had rehearsals at 2 a.m. on the days leading up to the announcement. I never really got into a good rhythm while I was there.

Paris was beautiful. Daniel Chaffey, owner of Reebok CrossFit Louvre, took me around to visit a handful of affiliates. I didn't really do the typical sightseeing thing, but I never do. It's not my style when I travel. On these trips, I want to see affiliates and do my job. That's about it. I do regret not seeing Notre Dame. I was reading *The Hunchback of Notre Dame* by Victor Hugo during the trip, and it was amazing. I recommend you put it on your must-read list.

My assistant on that trip was Jessica Sanki, a French CrossFitter who lived in Paris. She was great. She was all business and didn't talk much, which I appreciate most of the time. I don't like working with people I feel I have to take care of. She did well at facilitating everything I needed to make the trip successful.

It was a very long day and night before the announcement. I expected to do rehearsal, go back to my room, take a nap and then wake up to do my standard routine before the announcement. But I ended up not getting the nap. I was busy all the way through. I did get my standard 20-minute run at around 12:30 a.m. in the empty hotel gym. During these runs, I listen to music, mostly loud rap, Lil Wayne or something like that, and I rehearse what I'm going to say during the show. I like to rehearse with distractions. I know that if I can get it clean with music blaring while running, I should have no problem doing it on camera in an hour or two.

An important piece to remember about this process for me: I only rehearse like this after I have completely figured out how I am going to do it. For the actual planning, I don't want distractions. I need quiet time to figure out how I want to make the announcement. I don't ever plan the actual announcements ahead of time. When traveling to the host city, often on the flight, I usually have a general idea of how I want to announce the test, but I never finalize it until I see the actual location. Once in that environment, I figure out the details of the announcement—how I want to do it, what I will incorporate into it, etc.

People would probably think it's silly if they knew how much thought I give to announcements that last anywhere from 30 seconds to 2 minutes, but they are that important to me. I want it done a certain way, and I want to do it right. I think of everything I'm going to say and the order I'll say it in. I give a lot of thought to when the info will be delivered and how. Once at the venue, I shut everyone out and do some more rehearsals. I do my last-minute walkthrough in my mind. About 5 minutes to the show, I walk out and do one or two more silent rehearsals in my head among the crowd. Then I get ready for the real streamed announcement.

At around 1:15 a.m., we arrived at the venue, which, thankfully, was a quick walk from the hotel. I was really surprised at how many people showed up at 2 a.m. They were a great crowd and super into it. Sam Briggs and Kristin Holte went head-to-head and absolutely crushed the test. I was very pleased to see them go first, and I was actually surprised at their times—they did it much faster than I expected. I expected it to be around 11-12 minutes for the best, but I was happily proved wrong. I also like how the test played out, how hard it was for them.

After the show, people at the gym stayed and did the test. We didn't end up leaving until about 3:30 or 4.

The next day I slept in, which was great, and then I was able to visit some of the Paris special-operations units that keep the city safe. That was fun, and I was able to get some shooting in on their indoor range.

I flew home Saturday. I was exhausted from the trip, but I started to pay close attention to the leaderboard and how everyone was doing. I really enjoy seeing the top scores. I also like to pay attention to the vibe around the test. People seemed to be into 17.1 and really liked it.

One thing I forgot to mention: About three or four weeks before announcing the first workout, I used Instagram to tease that you would need 50- and 35-lb. dumbbells. I did not expect the negative backlash that followed. I thought people would be excited to know there was a new piece of equipment in the Open and they had time to prepare. Boy, was I wrong. People took to social media to complain like crazy. But what's funny is that most of the loudest complainers were not even affiliate owners. We did have some complaints from affiliate owners, but overall they were very supportive.

The inclusion of the dumbbell was the right move at the right time, and I am very happy we did it. The dumbbell will be included in future editions of the Open.

As for my go with 17.1, I wasn't pleased with it. I had done it a few times in testing, but I did it in my garage, where I only had a 45-lb. dumbbell. I actually did it before getting on the plane to fly to Paris for the announcement, and that left my back sore for days. For my actual attempts, I like to do them in the official Open window to be legit. I did 17.1 on Saturday, and I was beginning to get sick. The 50-lb. dumbbell made a huge difference. I got crushed. I had hoped to get close to finishing, but that was not the case. I did two or three burpees on the final set. The dumbbell felt so heavy.

At the end of Week 1, I was happy with how 17.1 had played out for the community as the first test of the 2017 season.

Random thought about the programming for the Games: wheelbarrow. Maybe it's time to use that again. Wheelbarrow and shovel.

17.2

COMPLETE AS MANY ROUNDS AND REPS AS POSSIBLE IN 12 MINUTES OF:

2 ROUNDS OF:

50 FT. OF WEIGHTED WALKING LUNGES

16 TOES-TO-BARS

8 POWER CLEANS

THEN, 2 ROUNDS OF:

50 FT. OF WEIGHTED WALKING LUNGES

16 BAR MUSCLE-UPS

8 POWER CLEANS

ETC., ALTERNATING BETWEEN TOES-TO-BARS AND BAR MUSCLE-UPS EVERY 2 ROUNDS.

MEN USE 50-LB. DUMBBELLS

WOMEN USE 35-LB. DUMBBELLS

17.2 was going to be the return of the dumbbell. A second theme: It was going to be a variant of 2016's lunge workout. In 16.1 we did overhead walking lunges with a barbell, and people were not happy about that. Small gyms had legitimate complaints. One issue was a lack of space to do the 25 feet out and back. Another was that lunging with a barbell overhead takes up even more space than lunging without a barbell. I wanted to program another lunge workout all gyms could do. The complaint this time was that people would need two dumbbells instead of one. I even heard stories of affiliate owners who purchased dumbbells for Week 1, returned them and then had to go out and buy them again.

This test went through a few iterations, too. The idea was to keep everyone in the game until the muscle-ups hit. At that point, the workout is essentially over for people who can't do a muscle-up—or they get their first muscle-up, which actually happens a lot in the Open. I'm OK if people hit a point where they can't advance in these events. It's a way of having tests that the best in the world and average Joes can do. Average Joes will be stopped while the best continue on. In designing the tests, the key is deciding when the average Joes are stopped. Last year, I put a stopping point right at the beginning of 16.3, the snatch/muscle-up workout, and I did that to send a message to the community: Work on these things. Get them. You and your clients can do them. You just need to make the movements a priority and believe that everyone can do them.

Another unique feature of this one: the low reps on the dumbbell cleans. The 8 cleans don't seem like much. The truth is they are an annoyance and contribute to the grip factor of the test.

Of note: The reps didn't change on the toes-to-bars and the bar muscle-ups. Traditional thinking would suggest the bar muscle-ups should perhaps drop down to 8 or 10. That's honestly how I would probably program it as a workout for a CrossFit group class. But I wanted to keep the reps the same for a few reasons. As I mentioned before, only some people can do a bar muscle-up. Of those who can, someone like me can get a few, but those who are really good will fly through. That's the point: The 16 reps would be a huge wall for those who are not highly conditioned next-level athletes, but they would not be a problem for others. The next-level athletes can shine in this workout, and shine they did.

The announcement in Columbus, Ohio, was fun and easy. We did it at the new Rogue Fitness Headquarters facility, which is amazing. I really enjoyed seeing it, and I'm proud of how far Rogue has come. Its growth is in large part reflective of our growth. As our community has grown, Rogue has been able to grow and be tremendously successful. Which leads us to the new 600,000-square-foot facility they were in the process of moving into in 2017.

When we were selecting locations for the 2017 Open announcements, I decided early on that the new Rogue facility would be one of our venues. Bill and I thought we could time the announcement around the grand opening, so we planned for that. They had some delays in construction and pushed back the grand opening, but we didn't change the date of the Open announcement—the same weekend of the Arnold Sports Festival, also in Columbus.

I hate the Arnold Sports Festival, trade shows and industry shows in general. I see their value for companies in those industries, but I am not a fan of having our teams work a booth. Years ago, I think in 2008, CrossFit decided to man a small booth at the SHOT Show, the largest trade show in the world for weapons, shooting and hunting. Greg wanted our booth to have a challenge, so we hosted the "*fastest Fran.*" I think we offered $5,000 to the person who could complete Fran faster than 2:30 or so. We didn't have many takers. I think the only one who gave it a go was a SEAL friend of mine who was a really good CrossFit athlete, but he tackled it hung over and didn't put in a great performance. Since then, I have hated trade shows.

So it wasn't a plus for me to have the freak show that is the Arnold in Columbus on the same weekend as the Open announcement. I was staying downtown and was able to avoid the show entirely and the mess that surrounds it, although I saw some huge bodybuilders in the gym stretching or preparing for a show when I was doing my routine pre-announcement 20-minute treadmill run.

Prior to this trip, I was having some sinus issues, and they continued. I have struggled with sinus issues over the years, and when I travel in blitz mode like I do during the Open and Regionals, I usually get hit. This year, after years of seeing an ENT and allergist, two surgeries and countless visits to doctors, I have seen improvement. Because I didn't feel good, I called my doctor and asked for some advice. He steered me in the right direction, and I felt better for the actual show. It reminded me of when we did the announcement in Boulder years ago. I was very sick, I couldn't sleep at night, and I was self-medicating.

The actual announcement went off fine in my eyes. I was happy with my piece, the show and the athletes' performances. Immediately following the show, I received texts from some athletes with regard to the grip on the dumbbell. This was the beginning of what would become an issue in the upcoming days. Our rule was that athletes must maintain a full grip on the dumbbell handle during the lunge. I didn't want athletes resting the dumbbell on their shoulders. But it turns out you can rest the dumbbells on your shoulders while maintaining a full grip on the handles. In hindsight, I think I should have addressed the issue then by saying you can't rest the dumbbells on your shoulders. But we didn't make that call, and I don't view this as a mistake. I think we stayed true to our rules, and that was fine. People maintained a full grip on the dumbbells, and some did that while resting them on their shoulders. Mat Fraser did not maintain a full grip, and that got him roasted on social media, so he redid the test.

I did 17.3 back in California on Saturday. I like to do the tests at home, not on the road. I was happy with my results: I made it back to the muscle-ups on the second round. In testing, I barely finished 1 round of muscle-ups before hitting the time cap.

17.3

PRIOR TO 8:00, COMPLETE:

3 ROUNDS OF:
6 CHEST-TO-BAR PULL-UPS
6 SQUAT SNATCHES (95/65 LB.)

THEN, 3 ROUNDS OF:
7 CHEST-TO-BAR PULL-UPS
5 SQUAT SNATCHES (135/95 LB.)

*PRIOR TO 12:00, COMPLETE 3 ROUNDS OF:
8 CHEST-TO-BAR PULL-UPS
4 SQUAT SNATCHES (185/135 LB.)

*PRIOR TO 16:00, COMPLETE 3 ROUNDS OF:
9 CHEST-TO-BAR PULL-UPS
3 SQUAT SNATCHES (225/155 LB.)

*PRIOR TO 20:00, COMPLETE 3 ROUNDS OF:
10 CHEST-TO-BAR PULL-UPS
2 SQUAT SNATCHES (245/175 LB.)

PRIOR TO 24:00, COMPLETE 3 ROUNDS OF:
11 CHEST-TO-BAR PULL-UPS
1 SQUAT SNATCH (265/185 LB.)

*IF ALL REPS ARE COMPLETED, TIME CAP EXTENDS BY 4 MINUTES.

17.3 was a really fun test. It was obviously influenced by 16.2.

16.2 RX'D

ON A 4-MINUTE CLOCK, COMPLETE AS MANY REPS AS POSSIBLE OF:
25 TOES-TO-BARS
50 DOUBLE-UNDERS
15 SQUAT CLEANS (135/85 LB.)

IF COMPLETED BEFORE 4:00, ADD 4 MINUTES AND PROCEED TO:

25 TOES-TO-BARS

50 DOUBLE-UNDERS

13 SQUAT CLEANS (185/115 LB.)

IF COMPLETED BEFORE 8:00, ADD 4 MINUTES AND PROCEED TO:

25 TOES-TO-BARS

50 DOUBLE-UNDERS

11 SQUAT CLEANS (225/145 LB.)

IF COMPLETED BEFORE 12:00, ADD 4 MINUTES AND PROCEED TO:

25 TOES-TO-BARS

50 DOUBLE-UNDERS

9 SQUAT CLEANS (275/175 LB.)

IF COMPLETED BEFORE 16:00, ADD 4 MINUTES AND PROCEED TO:

25 TOES-TO-BARS

50 DOUBLE-UNDERS

7 SQUAT CLEANS (315/205 LB.)

STOP AT 20 MINUTES

I thought 17.3 was an improvement on and a very good variant of 16.2. I say improvement because 16.2 created an issue when a ton of people couldn't get past the first section. Their event was over in 4 minutes. In 17.3, the opening set was 8 minutes for everybody, regardless of fitness level. The 2017 test also involved 3 rounds of work before advancing, whereas 16.4 required only 1 round of work. The first version I created in the early stages of 17.3 involved a single round of work before advancing, just like 16.2. But it didn't feel balanced. This was the initial design:

21 PULL-UPS

21 SQUAT SNATCHES (95 LB.)

24 PULL-UPS

18 SQUAT SNATCHES (135 LB.)

27 PULL-UPS

15 SQUAT SNATCHES (185 LB.)

ETC.

In the original version, the pull-ups really become the *"easy"* part of the test. You knock them out and then grind on a large set of snatches.

The next evolution included 2 sets, but I finally decided on the 3-set variant so athletes moved back and forth and the work felt more balanced.

In tests like this, it's challenging to get the loading right for the top athletes. I think I got this one right. It was *"lighter"* overall than 16.2, and I base this on the number of people who were able to finish the workouts. About 30 males finished 16.2, and about 200 men finished 17.3. On the women's side, I actually made 17.3 a little stiffer compared to 16.2, and the test was more appropriate because of that.

We did the announcement in San Antonio, Texas. I enjoyed hanging out with Mat Fraser, Scott Panchik and Cole Sager. I like those guys. I like being with the boys and giving them a hard time—especially Mat. Mat's a strong-willed guy and a fierce competitor. I enjoy pushing their buttons and seeing where I can get them to crack—just ask Rich Froning or Dan Bailey.

My announcement, and how I used the whiteboard, was a highlight for me. It was very confusing when I introduced 17.3, and that's exactly how I wanted it to play out. The numbers were all over the map, but they made perfect sense to me, and they suited the workout. During the announcement, I took the audience through a quick explanation but only those who were paying very close attention would know exactly what was going on.

I really had no idea if 17.3 could or would be completed under the time cap. I didn't have athletes who could complete it in testing. I just had my experience in programming these tests. I thought people would be able to complete it, and I wanted that to happen, so I was very nervous as I watched it play out. I was wondering if they could complete it and essentially provide proof of concept. Mat not only finished it but also posted one of the fastest times in the world even though he was one of the first people to do it.

A very special moment: seeing Cole hit one snatch at 265 lb. after missing 4 times. I didn't think he was going to get that lift, but I was very proud of him when he did.

I did 17.3 twice between the time it was announced and the submission deadline. The first time I got 1 snatch at 135 lb. and missed 2. The second time I finished 1 round at 135. I was pleased to get through 1 round of 135. The squat snatch is one of my worst movements, with handstand push-ups being another.

17.4 (16.4)

COMPLETE AS MANY ROUNDS AND REPS AS POSSIBLE IN 13 MINUTES OF:

55 DEADLIFTS

55 WALL-BALL SHOTS

55-CALORIE ROW

55 HANDSTAND PUSH-UPS

MEN DEADLIFT 225 LB. AND THROW A 20-LB. BALL TO A 10-FT. TARGET

WOMEN DEADLIFT 155 LB. AND THROW A 14-LB. BALL TO A 9-FT. TARGET

17.4 was our required repeat workout. Of course when I say "*required*," nobody is holding us to that. We could easily not repeat a workout, but I believe that would be a step in the wrong direction. Repeat workouts are a fundamental part of the CrossFit program and methodology. Redoing workouts lets us monitor progress and growth. Repeating workouts lets us know if our program is actually working or not, and providing an opportunity for that evaluation has always been a big part of my Open programming. I also like to apply that principle to the other stages of the competition, but I don't always stick to it when designing Regionals and the Games. There is an assumption that we will announce a repeat workout in every Open and it's just a matter of which one is repeated. This year I decided 16.4 would be our repeat.

I made the decision while I was creating the other Open tests. I had a handful of good repeats that were on my list for this year, and I knew what

17.5 was going to be. After I created some of 2017's other Open tests, it just fell in place that 16.4 would fit nicely as the repeat.

I personally enjoy this test for what it represents. It's a classic chipper. A chipper is a workout that has you moving from one movement to the next and "chipping" your way through the reps—usually a lot of them. 17.4/16.4 opens with a heavy-ish deadlift at 225 lb., then goes to the wall-ball shot, which is a nice squatting movement to complement that heavy pull. Rowing provides another hip-opening movement but uses a different range of motion and requires a small pull. The sequence ends with handstand push-ups (HSPU).

Everything before the final movement is very doable for 99 percent of the people in the Open. But then we tack on the HSPU. This allows people to do a lot of work to get to the fourth movement, and if they don't have the ability to do high-rep HSPU, they'll stay there until the time cap. Had I created this one with HSPU earlier in the test, the movement would have stopped a lot of people and prevented them from doing the other work.

For the regular people of the world, most of them get to the HSPU and try to do as many as they can. For the best in the world, it's a matter of doing all the HSPU and getting into the second round. All the top athletes were capable of that.

We announced 17.4 from Mexico City, Mexico. I really enjoyed making the trip down there. It was my first time visiting the city and my first time in Mexico since I was young. When I was a child, my parents would take me to the bullfights in Tijuana. I remember seeing broken glass embedded in the walls of the arena to prevent people from climbing over. I eventually saw that sort of barrier again as an adult in Afghanistan, and I saw it again on this trip to Mexico City. For some reason, I've always been fascinated by that crude yet highly effective construction technique with built-in security.

I don't remember one trip to Mexico as a child. I was told my grandparents kidnapped me and took me there. My grandparents from my dad's side of the family apparently loved me so much that they decided they wanted to take me away from my parents and down to Mexico without permission. My parents were able to get me back without much incident, but again, I was too young to remember any of this. I just heard the stories years later.

I was able to visit a handful of affiliates in Mexico City. I was very impressed by the boxes and the people's enthusiasm for CrossFit. CrossFit culture was thriving in those gyms, and it's always great to see how big the brand is overseas. The city is one of the biggest in the world, and the pollution was noticeable. But I still enjoyed Mexico City and ate some great food.

Our announcement at Cygnus CrossFit went off great. It was a smaller production without all the lights and the big team that we normally bring in. We wanted to do a smaller show by design because the box we used was not very large and we were traveling internationally. But I really enjoyed that announcement and its style of production because everything was on a smaller scale.

The workout was a pain to remember for that announcement. I knew I wanted to announce all the other workouts we've repeated, and I asked Stephane to make me a list of what they were. I came up with a plan for how I was going to mention all of them, and then I had to memorize the script. I rehearsed that one a lot. I rehearse them all a lot, but this one in particular had so much info, and I couldn't risk fucking it up. I was able to get it right, and I was happy with how it came off.

Finally, I had a couple of interesting travel experiences on this trip. On my way in, I was waiting to board at LAX when an airport official walked a group of seven or eight people to the front of the line and allowed them to get on the plane first. I had no idea who they were, but by the looks of them I figured they were some young pop band or something like that. They acted and dressed like they were young stars who were getting the special treatment, but I had no clue who they were.

They boarded, then I boarded. And of course we were all sitting near each other. As I was placing my luggage into the overhead bin, I heard an "ouch" from one person and then "you should apologize to him" from another.

I looked to my left and saw the young blond boy of the group rubbing his head. To the right was the person who had demanded the apology.

"Apologize for what?" I quipped.

"You hit him in the head."

"I don't think he knows he did that," said one of the young ladies with the group.

I turned to the young man: "*I am sorry for accidentally bonking you in the head even though I didn't know that happened.*"

"*It's cool, mate,*" the kid replied in a strong Australian accent.

As we took our seats I tried to figure out who they could be. One of the girls was teaching the blond Aussie how to say basic words in Spanish.

"*That's how you would say you are the Red Ranger,*" she explained.

I had recently seen "*John Wick: Chapter 2,*" and during the previews I saw a trailer for a new Power Rangers movie. I Googled the new version and identified the young group sitting around me as the cast of that movie. I heard it did OK at the box office.

My departure from Mexico was a nightmare. The night before my flight, the restaurant we were dining at caught on fire, and we had to evacuate. As I was driving to the airport the next morning, I remember wondering if I had everything I needed. I was confident I did. Ninety percent of the time I don't check bags when I travel, so I checked in and got my boarding pass via an unmanned kiosk. No checked bag, no need to go to the counter.

I headed through security and bought some airport gifts for my family. I had plenty of time to relax, so I bought a hamburger to go and then got in line to board. At that point I saw Jimi Letchford come up to the gate, and he looked out of breath. Jimi is a longtime employee of CrossFit Inc. and a friend. He's a former U.S. Marine who wrestled at the Naval Academy, and he looks like a pit bull. A nice pit bull.

"*What's going on, Jimi?*"

"*Man, I just had to go through this huge ordeal because I forgot to bring my customs slip with me.*"

"*What do you mean 'customs slip?'*"

"*They give you this card when you come in the country, and you need it on your way out. When you exit, you present it to the flight crew and they let you board. If you don't have it, you have to go through this huge process to get it, and it took me about an hour.*"

"*Oh, shit.*"

"*You don't have your customs card?*"

*"Nope."*

I was not looking forward to this adventure. I now needed to get a customs card, and my flight was boarding in a few minutes.

They give you these little customs cards when you land, but I didn't hear anyone make a big deal about keeping it or having it when you come back to the airport. And recall that I didn't go to a counter to check in with someone. I assume I would have been asked for the card there, too. But I didn't have it, and my flight was boarding in two minutes.

I went up to the counter and told the guy I didn't have my customs card. He basically said I will miss the flight because I don't have enough time to get a new one and return to board. I was beyond disappointed. I didn't want to spend the day in the airport waiting for the next flight. I just wanted to be on my way home. I asked what I had to do to get a new one, and I also offered to pay him if he would just let me on—but that didn't work either. He said I had to go to the customs office.

I told Jimi I was going for it and would try to make it back.

*"Sorry, man. See you back in the States."*

He had zero confidence that I could get it in time, and I had little confidence. I walked briskly away from the counter and down the terminal. After about 10 seconds, I made a decision. If I want this to happen, I need to do what I hate doing and what I judge people for: I need to run through the airport. I have always hated seeing people do that. Personally, I would rather just miss my flight than run through the airport. But not today, and not in Mexico City. I wanted out, so I ran, and I ran fast.

The first thing I did while running was toss the hamburger I was carrying in a plastic container. Then I continued to run down the terminal to an intersection. I sprinted left toward the customs office and arrived within minutes. I went in huffing and puffing. Mexico City is about 7,300 feet above sea level, and I was feeling it. I asked for help, and the customs officials had me start on the paperwork. A few other people looked like they were in the same situation. I filled out all the paperwork and realized I would have to go through security again to get back to the terminal. Damn it.

Once the paperwork was filled out, they gave me a slip and told me to take it to the bank to pay. I couldn't pay there. I had to go somewhere else. What a racket.

The bank was down the hall, down the escalator to the right and down another hall. Unbelievable. I left the customs office and sprinted to a bank near the entrance to the airport. There was a line, and the girl attending the line said I could pay the fee at another small bank across the hall. So I ran across the hall and walked up to the window.

*"Five hundred pesos, por favor."*

I handed over my credit card.

*"We don't accept credit card. Cash only."*

I handed them American cash.

*"Pesos only."*

I was devastated. I suddenly felt I had no chance to make my flight. I turned to the other folks in the room and asked if anyone had pesos to exchange for U.S. dollars. Everyone looked at me like I was crazy.

One of the customers suggested I use my debit card, but when I handed the teller my card, the customer clarified things: *"I meant you need to go to the ATM and get money."*

Of course, the ATM was in another area of the airport.

I was done. I was going to miss the flight, damn it.

*"Hola. Are you Dave Castro?"*

It felt like an angel had appeared.

I truthfully don't even remember seeing this gentleman in the room before that.

*"Yes, I am! Please give me 500 pesos. I will give you cash."*

He said OK and pulled the money out. I handed him a wad of U.S. cash and paid without having to leave the line. In that frantic process, the man asked if he could get a picture. I said yes, of course, but he said we couldn't do it in the bank. So I finalized my payment, walked outside, snapped a quick photo with this savior from above and then sprinted back to the customs office. Customs did their thing and took longer than I wanted, but I had my new card. I actually made it through security quickly but was still a few hundred yards away from my gate, so I started running.

*"Final boarding call for Aeromexico Flight 186. David Castro, if you are in the boarding area, this is your last chance to board. This is your last chance to board."*

Those words were painful to hear, yet they gave me a tiny bit of hope. I knew I still had a chance—but a slim one. As I was sprinting down the terminal I saw my gate. The entire boarding area was empty except for the three flight attendants. They did not look happy. I gave them my slip and they let me on the plane. As I boarded, I saw Jimi again. I had seen him about 15 minutes before starting my adventure, and he looked at me as if he had seen a ghost.

*"I thought for sure you were going to miss the flight. How did you make it?"*

*"Jimi, I ran. I just ran."*

I did 17.4 a few days later in the U.S., and I didn't do too great. I got a few HSPU, but not a lot. I'm really bad at handstand push-ups.

17.5

10 ROUNDS OF:

9 THRUSTERS (95/65 LB.)

35 DOUBLE-UNDERS

I had played around with the final Open workout early in the process of programming the Open. I knew I didn't want to pair thrusters with pull-ups because we've done that a few times. I wanted to try something different, so I went through different iterations on the whiteboard. I finally fell on thrusters and double-unders. I didn't want the weight to be heavy or the reps to be super high, but I wanted the workout to hurt. I played with various round and rep combos and settled on the final prescription. I liked 9 thrusters because that's the number of reps of the final round of Fran, and 10 rounds of 9 produce 90—essentially double Fran's thruster work. For the double-unders, 35 is not incredibly high, but it's a number that requires you to stay composed and focused. This one would bite, and it would bite hard. That's what I was looking for with the final test of the 2017 Open.

This announcement took place in Madison. It was going to be a dual-purpose trip: Do the announcement in the Games' new host city and visit the Alliant Energy Center to work on the Games. This plan worked out great and provided a boost of excitement and energy to the people and affiliates of Madison and Wisconsin. They really enjoyed hosting the Open announcement, and it gave them a small taste of what they could look forward to in August.

My announcements of the final workouts are generally much shorter. It's the end of the Open, and it's a straightforward test, so the announcement needs to be as concise as possible. The test speaks loudly, so I don't have to. It was going to be a short announcement, so I decided to up my game with my outfit. I wore a very nice Louis Vuitton suit made by an Italian bespoke tailor I sometimes use in downtown San Diego.

Moments after making the announcement, I walked up to Mat Fraser, who was in attendance. He made two comments that made me laugh. He thought the workout was too short and should be 20 rounds. Can you imagine 20 rounds of that? Twenty rounds might be appropriate for Games athletes, but probably not. And it would be a bit excessive for the rest of the world. Either way, it wouldn't be the sprint test I wanted. But I found it funny that that was one of Mat's first comments on the final test.

His second comment was that he thought the top 20-40 athletes in each region would tie. He didn't think there would be enough of a spread. I told him to trust me and watch. For the entire weekend I actually monitored the leaderboard closely, and once all the scores were collected, I sent him some screen shots of the leaderboard to prove his statement wrong. His reply was appropriate:

*"Yeah, I guess you really do know what you are doing."*

I was impressed with Sara Sigmundsdottir and Katrin Davidsdottir in Madison. I was surprised at how fast they went—they actually posted times that were faster than I thought we would see. But I was still pleased with the results of 17.5.

CrossFit Games Update Show host Rory McKernan and Adrian Bozman went head-to-head on 17.5 to finish their annual battle. They had me laughing because they went out so hot. They had finished 5 rounds in under 5 minutes and were killing it. Then the workout hit them hard and they slowed down a lot. Boz was around 11:30, and Rory was about a minute behind.

My experience was actually very similar. I set a pace I wanted to maintain, then I hit a wall and it got so hard. My time ended up in the high 16 minutes. I didn't redo this one. It hurt too much, and I was too sore for days.

*Friday, May 5, 3:51 p.m.*
Today I was looking at the schedule and format. I think I can reduce the size of one of the outside competition areas. This is a huge shift in focus and planning. I'm thinking the north lot will have just one field of play: the obstacle course. If I took out the 10-lane floor that we planned to have next to the O-course, I think I could get everything done in the dog park. It would probably mean no Big Bobs, but that's actually OK.

I will dig into this some more. My team will hate this large shift in planning.

*4:05 p.m.*
I have created a copy of my original schedule, and I'm butchering the current plan. I wasn't happy with it, and I think it can be better. Oh well, here we go. This is Games planning at its finest—change after change.

*Saturday, May 6, 4:40 p.m.*
Today I went to Troy CrossFit's grand-opening party, a quick visit to support a friend of mine, Hector Cabrera. On the ride home from that visit it started pouring rain. I was riding my Harley, and the rain actually felt pretty good. I didn't mind it.

This afternoon, while watching the Kentucky Derby, I decided to work on the schedule. I have continued to make a lot of changes. I'm still trying to see if the new plan works. Basically, I'm moving more things onto the same courses on the same days. Doing so will make the fan experience a little more manageable, but something has to give. Every year, some of my ideas are deleted or put away for other years just because of timing and the schedule. Right now, I'm at the stage where I have to delete an event for the masters. Working on that now.

In terms of the Team competition: I've made a big decision to have them in the water only once. I had thought about putting them in the water twice, as I planned to do with the individuals, but now it's looking like that's only going to happen once, too.

In terms of the individuals, I am making them start the weekend off with three events. This will provide a good wake-up call, and they'll find out right away who is there to compete and who is there to participate.

*Sunday, May 7, 2:42 p.m.*

I just had a great idea: make an 800-meter run course off the north-lot floor that I was thinking about killing. This actually solves a lot of my problems and would make that venue more useable and valuable. I'm going to work on that right now—and watch the Cavs game, too.

*6:21*

I worked on the schedule and watched the basketball game. LeBron and the Cavs are good.

I like where the schedule is going. I sent a note to Johnny Mac to figure out the 800-meter run course, and I sent a note to Pat to let him know the schedule is going through some major changes.

Johnny said he was out at the venue earlier and had a good day testing the bike course. He's an avid cyclist, so I tasked him with creating a course and format for the individuals. He rode a course he thinks will take 10-11 minutes per lap. With that time frame, I would think two laps, maybe three. Not more. Trek is sponsoring the event and supporting us with some mountain bikes. We did a bike event once before, but those bikes were single speeds, and it was during the Camp Pendleton triathlon. This year, we'll use Trek mountain bikes, and they will have gears. It's going to be interesting to see how the athletes respond to that. Overall, I think the bike event is a great addition to the Games.

I have ideas for next year's event, too, with regard to bikes. But this will be published before the 2018 competition, so I can't talk about that here.

*Monday, May 8, 1:37 p.m.*

I came into Yarrow today to program, and I was drawing a blank. I couldn't think of where to start or what to do. After looking at my computer for a few minutes and doing nothing, I decided to look at the schedule I've been working on for the past few weeks, but I didn't get anywhere on that, either. I decided to dive into an actual event instead. I broke out the pads of paper and pencils and started sketching things out. I normally use the computer for the schedule, and for programming I rely heavily on pencil and paper or the whiteboard.

I decided to tackle the weightlifting event for individuals. They're going to do a clean and jerk on one day and a snatch on another day. That's decided. Now I need to figure out what that will look like.

For the past few years at the Games the *"heavy weight"* has been included in sprint ladders, and I was very happy with how those played out. Those were great events to watch and compete in. But in my mind they need a break—at least for this year. So we're going to go to a more conventional lift.

*(I just had an idea while writing this: Maybe one day is conventional and the second is ladder style. I'll come back to this idea later.)*

I want to have platforms for each athlete and rotate through so each lifts alone—much like we did three years ago with the overhead squat. In that one, Rich was able to tie Mat on his lift, and then he *(and Tommy Hackenbruck)* went for 400 lb. but missed.

I want to use that format again, but with a twist: The top lifters will qualify for another round. We've never used this format before. Everyone will get three lifts, and the top 12 will advance and get two more lifts as they compete against each other in the same heat. I have to figure out how to make this work with timing and the schedule, and it can't take all day. I have to play with a lot of numbers and time variations.

It will help if I can get 20 platforms on the field of play. That's what I'm planning on now, and if it's doable, I'll have two athletes lift at a time for the first heats involving everyone. It's not as ideal as one at a time, but it's much better than having everyone go at the same time, which we have done often in the past, especially at Regionals. It's just really hard to keep track of what's going on and who is doing what.

*(I'm still thinking about the ladder idea. One problem with that: We did the ladder last year at the Games with the deadlift, so maybe I won't use this format. Still processing.)*

With the current schedule, I was able to get all of one gender's work done in 60 minutes—as long as we can get 20 platforms per heat. If we can't, it's back to the drawing board. At present, that's 60 minutes for one gender and two hours for both.

Making progress got my creative juices flowing, and I started looking at the same event for the teams. Events like this are challenging due to the sheer numbers of athletes: 40 teams of 6. But it needs to be done, and I'm making progress on a setup.

All three male or female members take a platform, and they have 7 minutes total for each to find a max lift. The teams with the highest totals advance to a round in which the athletes lift solo.

I really want a spotlight—an actual light—on the individuals as they lift, and on the teams when it's their turn. I'm pressing my crew to make sure that happens.

For now, I think I need to step away and reset. I've been at it for almost two hours, and I'm happy with what I accomplished.

Another thing: In the past 12 hours, I have released Day 1 of Regionals for the individuals. So far it seems like people are excited. This evening I will release Event 3. Rich texted me to ask when I'm going to announce team events. I said, "*Before Regionals.*"

*7:44 p.m.*

I just saw another video of an affiliate that has Assault AirRunners, and there are some Regional competitors training on them. Man, Roger is frustrating me on this one. He told me he wasn't going to give them to any athletes, but he has given them to gyms the athletes have access to. In hindsight, I should have had him sign something, but I thought I could trust him.

*Tuesday, May 9, 12:05 p.m.*

I was driving to the shooting range and I had an idea for an interval-based test at the Games with built-in rest. We have never done that, and it might be time to give it a go. I was thinking maybe 2 or 3 rounds of interval work, and then X reps in the final round—so the last section is an actual race to completion.

That's the reason not to do AMRAPs and interval workouts in competition: You usually don't see a race to the finish line. You just see work being done, which isn't super exciting. The race makes the work exciting.

I like this idea. I just need to play it out a little, see where it goes. I'll take it to pencil and paper.

*Wednesday, May 10, 9:18 a.m.*

Just had a split-snatch idea: I want to bring the split snatch back to the Games. Could do a complex. Split snatch left, power snatch, split snatch right. I like it.

*Thursday, May 11, 10:02 a.m.*

Over the past couple of days I have largely been involved in posting the clues for the Regional workouts and posting the actual workouts.

I haven't done much work on Games stuff other than looking at the schedule a little more and laying it out on the whiteboard for teams and individuals. Now I'll use this layout as a checklist for things I need to do as I schedule and actually create workouts. I label the blocks on the board with "CF" where I need to create actual CrossFit workouts. Any slot that says CF is vacant at present, but that's where a typical CrossFit event will go.

People often complain that the Games are all odd things and outside-the-box tests, but I go out of my way to make sure we test plenty of pure CrossFit events. People just ignore that and focus on the tests the athletes were not prepared for.

*11:20 a.m.*

I just transferred my current global schedule into a traditional schedule that I use when I program the Games. There are huge differences between the two. One is more of a placeholder for times, largely to help me coordinate with the other events going on during the weekend, and the new one includes details of how the events will run. At this stage, I'll start working off the detailed schedule primarily. I already have some good ideas for events and the overall flow. Big Bob with body armor and a litter carry? Big Bob solo? Just stuff like that. It's actually better to do Big Bob solo because I can run quicker heats and get that part of the competition done and out of the way. If I do it as part of a big event, it will take much longer.

Big Bob takes up so much room. If I do a Big Bob/litter-carry event, it's four heats of 10. But, if I do a litter event with no Big Bob, I could have all 40 teams go at the same time—or even 20 and 20 in two heats.

I also found out 10 minutes ago from Justin that I wrote last night's Team Event 2 wrong on the Instagram announcement. That pisses me off. Darn it. I hate making mistakes like that, especially simple ones that shouldn't happen. It's all about attention to detail. I preach that and expect my people to pay attention to the details, but I missed this one. I'm frustrated about it but can't dwell on it. In the larger scheme of things it won't matter too much.

But I hate that I did that.

*3:13 p.m.*

Working on some of the actual event details now, creating workouts. This is where it gets fun and I get to be creative. I just had a Starbucks Nitro Cold Brew and I'm kinda bouncing all over the place. Sketching things out all over the whiteboard and my notepads.

I had a couple of thoughts. One on the O-course. What if we started with a SkiErg component? Have them SkiErg 20-30 calories to gas them out, then have them go through the O-course. That would be very unique to us and a cool expression of fitness. I will play more with that idea.

For the teams, I'm working on a Big Bob event. I came up with something that might be fun to do. I call it the Big Bob Beatdown: 1 minute on, 1 minute rest, 5 rounds. Push Big Bob for distance. It's a crazy interval-based test that would hurt.

In writing this, I just came up with another expression of it, something similar to the interval format I mentioned earlier for individuals: 4 rounds to push as far as you can in the minute, but then in the final round you have 2-3 minutes to push it all the way across the finish line. So in the final interval, teams will start in front of each other based on how far they pushed in the early rounds. This can be cool. And the best part of this version is that it ends with the Big Bob reset, which is key. In a lot of these events, it's very time consuming to reset the gear for the next heats.

*4:27 p.m.*

I was going through the schedule and time blocks and putting some movements on the board. While doing that, I came across something that I liked, the combo of the GHD and a snatch complex.

I was thinking GHD sit-up, barbell power snatch left leg, center, right leg, for 3 or 4 rounds. But then I switched direction and thought, "*Well, I could make it a combo of barbell and dumbbell.*"

Something like 45 reps on the GHD, 18 left-arm snatches with a dumbbell (*left leg, center, right leg*), then 45 GHD reps, then 18 right-arm snatches with a dumbbell (*left leg, center, right leg*), then 45 GHD reps, then barbell snatches (*left leg, center, right leg*).

I like where this is going. I'll obviously have to test the shit out of it, but it's a start. Actually, it's the first true CrossFit event—besides Amanda—that I have really programmed for this year's Games.

Yes, this is how it always happens. The Games are just a few months away, and the CrossFit tests are only now coming together.

Overall, I put in a lot of time and had some good sessions today. I feel happy with where today ended up.

*Sunday, May 14, 10:14 a.m.*
I had a very productive brainstorming session this morning. I came up with a few workouts that will be butchered and changed over the course of testing with real athletes in the coming months. I want to include a sprint-style workout with bar muscle-ups, heavy deadlifts and overhead squats (OHS). And a HSPU/sled push (*but maybe a yoke walk*).

I also came up with a few crazy requests I texted to Bill Henniger.

*"Can you make a small calf that they can carry?"*

*"Can you make a cheese-like object to carry, lift, throw, etc."*

At this point, I find myself drifting to Team ideas, but I'm forcing myself to focus on the individuals only.

On that note, Bill suggested by text a tug of war for the Team competition. We did tug of war before—during the Tahoe Throwdown—and it was a huge success. We all really enjoyed it. Since then, we have always wondered if we should include tug of war. We have never included it in the Games, but I feel comfortable this year playing with the idea. I just need some time to think about it and play with the concept of actually doing it. We will see.

I also came in worrying I was doing too many long endurance tests this year, but I'm confident we are not. It's just enough. At some stage in my process, I really dive into the actual analysis of the Games weekend, and I take a detailed look at all the time domains and how that distribution looks across all tests.

*Monday, May 15, 4:35 p.m.*

Today I received the big barricades Bill suggested we use in the event where athletes throw a med ball over the wall and then burpee over the wall. This was an early concept I was playing with and planning on using. I'm looking at the barricades now, and I think they have the potential to work great. They are the plastic center dividers you see on roads. You fill them with water to add the weight. They look rough. We might have to dress them up a little, put some signage on them and maybe put something across the top to soften things a little. But the heights are great, and with some water in them they will be super stable.

Another cool thing happened today. Justin had sent me an email a few days ago about the Team Series. He had asked me to look at it, but I forgot. I came across it today and took a close look. Basically, Megan Mitchell, an old-school CrossFit HQ employee who works on our Games team, suggested a complete overhaul of the Team Series. Instead of teams of four and multiple weeks of competition, she suggested a pairs competition over the course of one or two weeks. The old model was three workout blocks over three weeks. So if you wanted to do a super team, it was actually really hard to make it happen. We then moved it to two weekends—which is better, but you still have to travel twice. With the new format, we could just make it one weekend.

I actually really like the idea of making the Team Series a pairs competition. It's one of the better ideas that's been suggested with regard to that competition. She suggested a few divisions—same gender and mixed gender. I almost think having separate competitions like that might be cool.

Changing the Team Series is not a problem for me. I like trying new things and challenging our current model. In the past, we have made some big changes to the Games and the Games season, and they always surprise people. With these changes, I can see the competitiveness and inclusiveness of the Team Series being much higher. Another big plus with this format would be programming for two instead of four athletes. Programming fun, hard events is so much easier with small numbers.

*5:58 p.m.*

I did some more work on the schedule, particularly Saturday. I think I overloaded that day, so I had to dive into it to find out how I am going to make events that fit. I pulled an Individual event out, but that might become a situation where we do one walk-out and two events. That little technique actually saves a ton of time in transitions and heats. Basically, the athletes take the floor and do two events instead of one. We haven't done it that often, and it's usually reserved for Sunday events, but this approach always makes for entertaining shows.

*Wednesday, May 17, 2:07 p.m.*
Today was all about the schedule. I really focused on tying it all together.

My original Friday was looking like this:

TEAM O-COURSE

INDIVIDUAL O-COURSE

TEAM SNATCH

INDIVIDUAL SNATCH

TEAM CF

INDIVIDUAL CF (MEDIUM-LONG)

INDIVIDUAL CF (SPRINT)

I didn't like how the flow felt, both for the show and for the test, so I played around with another variant:

TEAM O-COURSE

INDIVIDUAL O-COURSE

TEAM SNATCH

INDIVIDUAL SNATCH

INDIVIDUAL CF (MEDIUM-LONG)

TEAM CF

INDIVIDUAL CF (SPRINT)

But after staring at the schedule and playing around with how it would play out, I decided on moving the medium-long Individual block and the

Team block before the heavy lifts. Everybody loves seeing the athletes go heavy, and those make great evening events. So I ended up with a schedule that looks like this:

**TEAM O-COURSE**

**INDIVIDUAL O-COURSE**

**INDIVIDUAL CF (MEDIUM-LONG)**

**TEAM CF**

**TEAM SNATCH**

**INDIVIDUAL SNATCH**

**INDIVIDUAL CF (SPRINT)**

I think it will make for a great layout on Friday. So for now, this is what Friday will look like. Now I actually need to program those events, but I have some good ideas flowing. I'll work on programming some of those tests while I travel for Regionals. I leave tomorrow for the first weekend of Regional competition.

*5:36 p.m.*

I just texted Bill to ask him how hard would it be to bring back the Banger—the sledgehammer event we used a few years back. I don't want to bring back the actual event but its pieces, specifically the low Banger, the one on the floor. I think it could make for an epic event.

*Thursday, May 18, 5:00 p.m.*

I am currently on a flight from Atlanta, Georgia, to Albany, New York. I land in about 20 minutes. From the airport I'll go straight to the venue. Once there, I'm going to watch Adrian give the athlete briefs for the first week of Regionals. I'm excited about the start of Regionals, but the truth of the matter is my head is in the Games right now. I know that when I get on the ground, the Regionals and this weekend's excitement will consume all my thoughts and energy.

The first weekend of Regionals is the most stressful. It's also the weekend where I'm most involved and pay the most attention. It's essentially the proof of concept for what we created—proof of concept for the schedule, the events, the flow, etc. After months of preparation and planning for eight events that have to be identical in eight locations over the course of three weeks, I get to see that the tests flow the way I designed them. I get to see that the tests were appropriate, or, sometimes, that they were not. I try to watch every aspect of the weekend and stay on top of the timing and the flow so we can make adjustments. Obviously, we cannot make adjustments to the actual tests, but we can change the layouts to increase spectator visibility, the spacing to increase athlete and judge safety, and hundreds of other small items like that. I also pay close attention to our broadcast and media streams, as well as our broadcasts and media streams from the other events on that weekend.

I like the venue in Albany. It's a large hockey arena. We used it last year for the Regional, and it's a good place to watch the show. I'm excited about going back to this one. I will be here for two days, and then I go to San Antonio, Texas, for the final day of the South Regional.

*Friday, May 19, 9:09 p.m.*
Day 1 of the Regionals is done. Overall, it was a good day. I was very happy with how the Team workouts played, and the Individual workouts went well.

One big surprise and disappointment: the pec injuries we had at the East Regional on the snatch/ring-dip event. In one of the early heats, I noticed a few guys stop and grab their chests. And then in the final heat, one of the guys who was giving Mat a run went down in pain. Once we saw this happen in the East, we gave the team at the South Regional a heads-up. They're a few hours behind us. We told them to let the athletes know what's going on so they can keep it in mind in when preparing strategy. One person at the South Regional went into the event with the injury already, and nobody else got injured in addition.

I've been involved in this sport for over 10 years, and here's a reality when people are competing at the highest levels: injuries happen. We have seen various types of injuries throughout the years, but to see four in one event in one day is really odd.

Injuries at this level of competition are not the norm, but they are a possibility when you have people pushing themselves to the limit as they race each other for points, for pride, for spots in the Games. People are more inclined to put themselves at risk in these events than they are in training.

I don't take injuries lightly. The last thing I want at this or any stage is injuries at our events. Whenever I see injuries at events, they put me in a somber mood.

CrossFit as a training methodology is extremely safe. We pride ourselves on mechanics, consistency and then intensity. Learn how to do the movements correctly, and then gradually increase the intensity over time. This process requires some self-monitoring and personal accountability, and if you combine that approach with a coach, CrossFit produces great results and is incredibly safe. I have been doing CrossFit for about 12 years and have not suffered any major injuries. I've had little tweaks here and there, but nothing torn, nothing pulled and nothing that required surgery.

When I think about the injuries at Regionals, I consider what I programmed and how much of it was programmed. Ninety reps—21-15-9 of both ring dips and snatches—are not outside what athletes are expected to perform. Then I take it back a little and think, *"Well, having them do that a few hours after performing Event 1, is that an issue?"* I honestly don't think so. The athletes always do multiple events at this stage—and these are the best in the world.

At this point, the issue might be that the athletes were not prepared. How often do you see athletes doing ring dips in training? I don't feel like it's very common these days. I think maybe we are exposing a weakness—a weakness that has led to injury for some. I have two more weeks to observe what happens. I don't think we will change the workout. That would be a knee-jerk reaction. Out of 40 athletes, four hurt themselves. So 36 had no issue, including people like Mat, Patrick Vellner and so on. And there were no injuries on the women's side at all.

On a brighter topic, I really enjoyed how the thruster/burpee workout played out and affected the Team athletes. I think I might take that one on to the Games—a more difficult version, of course.

*Saturday, May 20, 9:17 p.m.*
I'm currently on a flight from Albany to San Antonio *(via Chicago)*. Two Regional days are done, and one remains. At this stage, I'm mostly happy with the events. I really like the inclusion of the Worm for the teams. It adds some fun stuff and really highlights teamwork.

Since I have some time on this flight, I'm going to talk about the programming of Day 1 and Day 2 of Regionals.

2017 CROSSFIT GAMES REGIONALS TEAM EVENT 1

MF PAIR 1 (EACH):

500-M RUN

24 STRICT HANDSTAND PUSH-UPS

24 DUMBBELL SNATCHES

MF PAIR 2 (EACH):

500-M RUN

28 STRICT HANDSTAND PUSH-UPS

28 DUMBBELL SNATCHES

MF PAIR 3 (EACH):

500-M RUN

32 STRICT HANDSTAND PUSH-UPS

32 DUMBBELL SNATCHES

MEN SNATCH 80-LB. DUMBBELL

WOMEN SNATCH 55-LB. DUMBBELL

ORDER: MF, MF, MF

TIME CAP: 25 MINUTES

This event is designed to highlight the strengths and weaknesses of each team member. It's an opportunity for each athlete to contribute an individual effort. In creating this one, I was actually working on it as six-person relay. One goes, then the next and so forth. But I would have had to use a super short, quick test to fit that format in the schedule. Early on, when I was programming Individual workouts, I had determined I could use 20 Assault AirRunners at once. So that influenced this event. I decided to have a male and female go at the same time even though they are not doing it together. That played out great, and I'm happy with how it worked. A few teams that had members struggle with handstand push-ups didn't make the cap, but most did.

Let's go back to the AirRunner for a second. Keep in mind that I program the Individual events first most of the time. Generally, this has to do with equipment logistics. The AirRunners and handstand walls were being used on Friday by the individuals, so logistics dictate that the teams use them, too. And because Individual equipment dictated that we have a running element and a body-weight element for the Team event, I wanted to add a loaded element for the teams. That ended up being the dumbbell snatch.

If the reps were the same for every team member, a test like this wouldn't require strategy. By having slightly different rep schemes for each pair, I built in a need for strategy. Each team had to decide where to plug in its pairs to get the best time. Overall, I was happy with this one and how it played out.

As I was watching this event in Albany, I saw how we were using the chess-piece lane marker. Every pair that advances moves its chess piece forward to represent where the pair is in the event. At one point, a team was done and the other teams were still on the course, so I decided to try having finishing teams lay their chess piece down. That would allow you to look at the floor and instantly see who was done and who was not. It worked great. We will carry that over to other events in which it makes sense.

## 2017 CROSSFIT GAMES REGIONALS TEAM EVENT 2

40 WORM THRUSTERS

40 WORM BURPEES

30 WORM THRUSTERS

30 WORM BURPEES

ORDER: FULL TEAM

TIME CAP: 15 MINUTES

Team Event 2 was the first Regional test involving the Worm. I was very excited about its inclusion. During our trip to Columbus for 17.2, Justin and I had a meeting with Bill to discuss equipment for Regionals. We were going down the list of items that they would have to ship. We talked about how GHDs are such large items to ship. They were not trying to dissuade me from including them, just stating a fact.

I asked Bill if we could pull the GHDs from the kit and use Worms instead. He said yes, and I was very, very excited about that. I love the Worms and what they represent. They are one of the few tools that demand full teamwork. Communication is critical, as well as strength, conditioning and all the other facets of fitness. The Worm really has the ability to break down teams—and it brings teams together. So finding out we could include them in the kit was a highlight for me.

Once determined that we were going to have Worms, I quickly decided on how I was going to format the Team events for the weekend. Each day, the second Team workout would involve the Worm.

Event 2, the first Worm event, actually wasn't the first one I programmed. That would be Event 6 on Sunday. For that one I knew I wanted to repeat the Games event that had 50 clean and jerks for time. So I plugged that in first and built the others around it, with consideration for the equipment already being used on each day of the Regional.

Event 2 was a simple couplet of thrusters and burpees. I really liked how it affected the athletes. They were blasted after this test, completely wasted and laid out on the floor. That was the desired effect. This combo was so appealing that it makes me want to carry it over to the Games. I might just do that—but a stiffer version appropriate for those teams that qualify for the Games.

I wasn't so happy with the visual aspect. A few things bothered me, such as the teams' staggered positions during the event—but that was a must because of how much room the burpees take. I also didn't like the fact that they did the thrusters and burpees in the same spot. I would have preferred them to move much more to show their positions in the reps, but obviously the floor at the Regionals isn't big enough to allow for all that movement.

2017 CROSSFIT GAMES REGIONALS INDIVIDUAL EVENT 1

WEARING A WEIGHT VEST:

1,200-M RUN

THEN, 12 ROUNDS OF:

4 STRICT HANDSTAND PUSH-UPS

8 CHEST-TO-BAR PULL-UPS

12 SQUATS

MEN WEAR A 20-LB. VEST

WOMEN WEAR A 14-LB. VEST

TIME CAP: 25 MINUTES

Event 1 for the individuals was another favorite of mine. I wanted to do something Murph-like, and a few months ago I asked Tom Davin from 5.11 Tactical if we could do vests at Regionals. Tom is the CEO of 5.11, an ex-Marine Corp officer and a solid guy all around. I don't think he has ever said no to a request that I have had, no matter how crazy it is.

Murph as written would not work at Regionals as I would like. Murph at the Games works because we run outside. We were going to run on the Assault AirRunner at Regionals, and it wouldn't be a good test or visual if they did all the work going out and then came back and ran again in the same place. So I decided to do something very similar to Murph, something essentially inspired by Murph.

I started with the run and selected handstand push-ups because they would be easier to judge than regular push-ups. I feel confident having our team judge regular push-ups at the Games, but it can get ugly at Regionals with less-experienced judges.

Next, I played around with a bunch of different rep schemes but settled on the final prescription. I think I could have programmed it a little longer. I had the time available. But it's still a great test, and I was happy with it. The visuals were great as they moved their chess pieces down the floor. As a fan, you could really see who was winning at a glance, and that's a big positive.

I was surprised at how fast guys did it. These athletes really are impressive.

I also can't remember another Individual Regionals event in which we had 20 athletes go at once. This was great for the fans. Instead of sitting through 4 25-minute heats for each gender, they only had to sit through 2 25-minute heats of each. As an organizer, that time saving allowed me to program everything we needed to do that day.

### 2017 CROSSFIT GAMES REGIONALS INDIVIDUAL EVENT 2

21-15-9 REPS OF:

DUMBBELL SNATCHES

RING DIPS

MEN USE AN 80-LB. DUMBBELL

WOMEN USE A 55-LB. DUMBBELL

TIME CAP: 6 MINUTES

Individual Event 2 was meant to be a sprint, and we accomplished that goal. It was obviously not meant to injure people. I have a lot of thoughts on this but haven't settled on a conclusion yet.

Here is the tricky part: Once warned, the athletes in the South had zero injuries. It sounds like one guy went into that event hurt already, and he made it worse by doing it, but everyone else was fine. So in the East, we had 4 of 40 athletes get injured on that event. In the South, not one of 50 athletes got a new injury. Of note, all this does not seem to be a problem for women.

Another interesting fact: We used this standard for ring dips three years ago at Regionals. A big difference here is the speed of this event. In the 2014 event, they had to do 50 reps in a chipper, and in this one they were working faster in the 21-15-9 format.

I wonder if they are just going so fast that they red-line and put themselves at risk for injury. Apparently so. I don't think this is a reckless test. I think there is just some combination of competition speed and not being 100 percent prepared for this movement—and perhaps there were pre-existing or related injuries.

Another way I like to view it: How many people were fine? In the East, 90 percent of the competitors had zero issues, and in the South 100 percent were fine.

I programmed this one to be fast, so I included two movements with fast cycle times. I also used a famous CrossFit rep scheme to give it a very classical look and feel. Later on in the programming process, I would be compelled to use the same pieces of equipment and the same format to create an entirely different version of the test. But we'll talk about that later.

2017 CROSSFIT GAMES REGIONALS TEAM EVENT 3

MM PAIR:

20-CAL. ASSAULT AIRBIKE (EACH)

50 SYNCHRO WALL-BALL SHOTS

20 SYNCHRO BAR MUSCLE-UPS

20-CAL. ROW

FF PAIR:

15-CAL. ASSAULT AIRBIKE (EACH)

50 SYNCHRO WALL-BALL SHOTS

20 SYNCHRO BAR MUSCLE-UPS

15-CAL. ROW

MF PAIR:

20/15-CAL. ASSAULT AIRBIKE (EACH)

50 SYNCHRO WALL-BALL SHOTS

20 SYNCHRO BAR MUSCLE-UPS

20/15-CAL. ROW

MEN USE A 30-LB. BALL

WOMEN USE A 20-LB. BALL

ORDER: MM, FF, MF

TIME CAP: 25 MINUTES

This test was difficult for the teams to finish under the time cap of 25 minutes. I think I saw half the teams cap at the East Regional. In the first heat, no team finished. In the second heat, maybe one or two teams finished. In the final heat, most of them finished. So maybe it was less than half. But this one really taxed the athletes. I was happy it hit them like a ton of bricks.

In years past, Team athletes rarely moved so much for such long periods. Often, events were just quick relay after quick relay. But this one—and most of the others this year—had them engaged more. And that's especially true of the Worm events.

In Team Event 3, I liked the 30-lb. wall ball. The load was actually programmed before I selected 30 lb. for the Individual men. As I said earlier, my head judges actually talked me out of 20-lb. balls for the individuals.

2017 CROSSFIT GAMES REGIONALS TEAM EVENT 4

6 ROUNDS OF:

30 WORM PUSH PRESSES

1 ROPE CLIMB, EACH

ORDER: FULL TEAM

CAP: 15 MINUTES

Team Event 4 was meant to highlight teamwork and individual weaknesses on rope climbs.

As I was typing this write-up of Team Event 4, I had an idea. We've done the short rope and we've done fat ropes. It came to me that maybe we need to try a rope transfer with shorter ropes each time. This is something we did when I was in the Navy on our water O-courses. Basically, you have one rope that's about the length of our current short rope. A few feet in front of it, you have another that's a little bit shorter, then another that's even shorter, and so forth. So you climb higher and farther out with each rope.

It's harder than it sounds, as you can imagine. It's basically a legless rope climb with the added challenge of covering some distance and negotiating the transfers.

Tomorrow, I'll have Bill start working on some mock-ups and prototypes.

Back to Event 4: Teamwork is critical, and communication is very important. I was happy with how it played out. It turned out to be another chaotic team Worm event, and it made for a great race.

2017 CROSSFIT GAMES REGIONALS INDIVIDUAL EVENT 3

100-FT. DUMBBELL OVERHEAD WALKING LUNGE

100 DOUBLE-UNDERS

50 WALL-BALL SHOTS

15-FT. ROPE CLIMB, 10 ASCENTS

50 WALL-BALL SHOTS

100 DOUBLE-UNDERS

100-FT. DUMBBELL OVERHEAD WALKING LUNGE

MEN USE AN 80-LB. DUMBBELL AND A 30-LB. BALL.

WOMEN USE A 55-LB. DUMBBELL AND 20-LB. BALL.

TIME CAP: 16 MINUTES

Individual Event 3 was supposed to be a medium-long chipper. Again, I feel like it could have been a tad longer. But overall I was happy with how it was performed.

As I mentioned above, this version originally had 20- and 14-lb. wall balls, but I'm glad we made the change. I also had a version including a handstand walk, but after playing around with a lot of options, I couldn't get it to be as clean as I wanted.

A highlight was watching Fraser at the East Regional. He put his dumbbell down about 30 feet in as Vellner was starting his lunges. Dylan Malitsky, our floor announcer at that event, shouted over the mic, *"Can Vellner overtake*

*Fraser?*" or something to that effect. Fraser, who was picking up his dumbbell, shook his head with a resounding no. That's the championship fight and spirit I love from Mat. He's always fighting and always wants to win. So far, he's won a lot.

## 2017 CROSSFIT GAMES REGIONALS INDIVIDUAL EVENT 4

60-FT. HANDSTAND WALK

10 TOES-TO-BARS

10 DOUBLE KETTLEBELL DEADLIFTS

60-FT. HANDSTAND WALK

12 TOES-TO-BARS

12 DOUBLE KETTLEBELL DEADLIFTS

60-FT. HANDSTAND WALK

14 TOES-TO-BARS

14 DOUBLE KETTLEBELL DEADLIFTS

60-FT. HANDSTAND WALK

16 TOES-TO-BARS

16 DOUBLE KETTLEBELL DEADLIFTS

MEN USE TWO 150-LB. KETTLEBELLS

WOMEN USE TWO 106-LB. KETTLEBELLS

TIME CAP: 11 MINUTES

I think I missed the mark with the layout for Individual Event 4. Too much crossing over itself for my taste. It ends with the deadlifts, and then you run to the finish line, likely passing people who are still doing handstand walks. It's not as visually appealing as I want our events to be. I could clean it up by putting the handstand walk between the deadlifts and toes-to-bars, so athletes would only approach the finish line as they got closer with the deadlifts. I still might. I need to bust out the floor plan and dig to see if I want to make the change.

As I think it through, a change would create other problems for flow and layout, so I probably won't change it—but I will still take a look at it.

I think a better version could have been this:

10 TOES-TO-BARS

30-FT. HANDSTAND WALK

10 DEADLIFTS

30-FT. HANDSTAND WALK

12 TOES-TO-BARS

30-FT. HANDSTAND WALK

12 DEADLIFTS

30-FT. HANDSTAND WALK

14 TOES-TO-BARS

30-FT. HANDSTAND WALK

14 DEADLIFTS

30-FT. HANDSTAND WALK

16 TOES-TO-BARS

30-FT. HANDSTAND WALK

16 DEADLIFTS, CROSS THE FINISH LINE.

To really understand why this would be better, you have visualize it or write it on a mock floor. This version would be an A+ event visually, while I give the actual event a C.

I don't get them right every time, but I do learn from them and get better at this.

*Sunday, May 21, 11:40 p.m.*

I spent the day at the South Regional in San Antonio. I got in late last night, at 11:30 p.m., and went straight to bed. I contemplated getting up early and working out, but because I wanted to hear the team briefs, that would have meant a 5:30 wake-up. I can do that, and I have done that, but there's no need to push myself at Regionals just to fit a workout in a schedule that's already super busy. So I got six hours of sleep instead of five. I prefer to get eight or nine hours every night, but I can function with less when needed.

Wow—the venue was impressive. It's the Alamodome, a football stadium that's only about 14 years old. The back-of-house, athlete village and volunteer areas were great. Vendor village was great, too—but the place is just way too big. The entire stadium dwarfed the competition. They added some bleachers to one side of the venue, but they were so low in pitch that they didn't really give spectators a good view.

Sounds like the Regional team really likes the venue. It was easy to work with, and the team wants to go back. If we do, we all have ideas on how to improve and make it better.

This event is always great. It has the feel of an international event because of the inclusion of the South Americans. Lots of South American, Central American and Mexican fans and athletes are in attendance, and they're all so great and enthusiastic. I really enjoy this Regional for that reason.

On that note, this Regional is so demanding on the fans and event staff. We have to create additional heats to handle all the additional teams and individuals, and it makes for very long days. I'm going to fix that this year. Giving South America its own Regional is one part of a my big plan to adjust the Regionals and the qualifying process. I gave it a little more thought today at the airport, and I think we will end up somewhere like this:

Australia

South America

Asia

Europe 1

Europe 2

U.S. regions, with changes to give us four or five

Each region will have two to three subdivisions in the Open that feed into the Regional. These are my initial thoughts. I need to do a lot of deep diving to create a final plan.

Before I talk about the Day 3 events, I should mention that I showed up to see Head Judge Todd Widman talking with an athlete. When they were done speaking, I asked Todd what had happened. He briefed the teams and then told me he and the staff were getting trouble from this guy. As he was telling me this, the same guy walked up to talk to Todd. I told Todd to take care of it and let me know if he needed my help. The guy ended up saying there would be no more problems. Todd is great at handling situations like that.

Here are the final few workouts of the Regionals:

2017 CROSSFIT GAMES REGIONALS TEAM EVENT 5

AS MMM THEN FFF TRIOS:

125 CHEST-TO-BAR PULL-UPS W/ TEAMMATE IN HANG

100 TOES-TO-BARS W/ TEAMMATE IN HANG

100 DUMBBELL OVERHEAD SQUATS

MEN USE AN 80-LB. DUMBBELL

WOMEN USE A 55-LB. DUMBBELL

ORDER: MMM, FFF

TIME CAP: 20 MINUTES

I enjoyed how this event played out. I originally tested it with a team that did 100, 100 and 100. That was too short. So I then created it at as 150, 125 and 100. We had our team test it during the video shoots, and it was way too long. After much deliberation with Stephane, Pat and Adrian, we decided to drop the reps. We reduced the reps on the pull-ups to 125 and on the toes-to-bars back to 100. To finish this event under the time cap, you really have to work hard—and we saw some teams do that.

I saw a couple of floor tweaks today that I am having the team implement just to improve the visual for the fans and the athletes. Nothing too major on this event.

### 2017 CROSSFIT GAMES REGIONALS TEAM EVENT 6 (FINAL)

### 50 WORM CLEAN AND JERKS

### ORDER: FULL TEAM

### TIME CAP: 10 MINUTES

The final Team event for this year's Regionals was the same as Worm Finale, the final Team event from the Games in 2015: 50 clean and jerks for time with the Worm.

I think I should have upped the reps. Teams really crushed this. They used a touch-and-go technique that was much faster than what teams were using at the Games two years ago. The Regional teams also had a chance to practice and prepare for this event, whereas I briefed it on the floor at the Games and gave the teams there only minutes to determine their strategy. As a Regional event, it was an appropriate test and a great finale. The fact that some teams did it in just over 4 minutes really impressed me, and I second-guessed the number of reps I had programmed. I wanted this test to be a tad longer, in the range of 5 or 6 minutes.

While I was watching this event, I thought of doing a Worm complex at the Games: clean, squat, push press to other side, squat, drop Worm, repeat.

It's essentially the same thing they did today but with a squat every time they get the Worm to their shoulders. That would be brutal. It might be fun to play with it in Madison.

### 2017 CROSSFIT GAMES REGIONALS INDIVIDUAL EVENT 5

### 21-15-9 REPS OF:

### MUSCLE-UPS

### SINGLE-ARM OVERHEAD SQUATS

### MEN USE AN 80-LB. DUMBBELL

### WOMEN USE A 55-LB. DUMBBELL

### TIME CAP: 11 MINUTES

Created toward the end of Regionals planning, Event 5 was obviously heavily influenced by Event 2. I wanted do something that used three identical components—same rep scheme, same dumbbell weight and same gymnastics apparatus—but I wanted the two tests to be very different.

Event 2 was a 21-15-9 all-out sprint that required little strategy. Event 5 was a 21-15-9 medium-length/long test that required smart pacing and a lot of thought.

In Event 2, they took the dumbbell from the floor to overhead in one violent movement. In Event 5, they used the same dumbbell, but we replaced the violence and aggression of the snatch with a movement that required precision and control: the single-arm overhead squat.

Event 2's rings were set low, and the athletes dipped fast and usually unbroken. In Event 5, the rings were set high for the more demanding and challenging ring muscle-up, which has a little dip in it, too, depending on where you finish in the transition from pull to push. Most athletes could not do the ring muscle-ups unbroken—especially the first set.

One other little tweak I made: Event 2 started with the dumbbell, and Event 5 started with the rings. Overall, I'm happy with how the tests turned out. Event 5 isn't the most exciting, especially in the lower heats, but it's a necessary test, and sometimes I need to compromise a little of the show to create a good test that complements the other aspects of the weekend.

## 2017 CROSSFIT GAMES REGIONALS INDIVIDUAL EVENT 6 (FINAL)

30/25-CAL. BIKE

20 BURPEE BOX JUMP-OVERS

10 SANDBAG CLEANS

MEN USE A 30-IN. BOX AND A 150-LB. BAG

WOMEN USE A 24-IN. BOX AND A 100-LB. BAG

TIME CAP: 6 MINUTES

This event was supposed to be a sprint. I think it mostly accomplished that.

After viewing it today, I was a little underwhelmed with the action it provided. I wanted to see more excitement, more drama. Maybe I need to see it from a better position. I probably should have gone down to the floor to see if it met my standards, but I watched it from another spot at the South Regional. I think Event 6 came out well and is still a good test, but I need some more convincing that it's a great test. I have two more weekends of Regional competition to figure that out.

Week 1 of Regionals is wrapped up, and I'm flying home for a few days of rest. Actually, that's not true. I'll work on Games programming for a few days before flying to Nashville on Thursday. I will be there Friday, and then I come back to San Diego for the Saturday and Sunday of the California Regional. Both of these events should be fun to attend.

*Monday, May 22, 5:42 p.m.*
I didn't do as much as I wanted to on the programming. I came into Yarrow for a one-hour session. I worked mostly on Friday's schedule again. I don't think it's going to work, so I had to really dig into the O-course events and come up with some realistic timing. I did a real schedule for the Individual O-course event and figured it would take an hour and 15 minutes to get one gender through an exciting bracket event, much like we did at Pendleton. I had originally allotted one hour. The original plan was to handle both genders in two hours, and now we need to find an additional 30 minutes. In a timeline that's already tight, another 30 minutes can be a game changer.

I then dove into a timeline for the teams. Their competition will not be a bracket. This new timeline has them going for 90 minutes. My initial assessment was 60, so I have an additional hour of time to account for. I think I'm going to start Friday at 8 a.m. with the teams at the O-course. Even with that, I still have a schedule that goes almost to 10 p.m. I am not aiming to end the day at 10 p.m.

I have the individuals doing four events: the O-course, two classic CrossFit events *(one long, one short)* and a snatch event. The teams are doing the O-course, a CrossFit workout and the snatch. Even with an 8 a.m. start, those seven events won't be complete until 10 p.m.

I think I found a solution: doing both CrossFit events for individuals in heats of 20. That's a lot of bodies on the floor, and it basically means no barbells. But we didn't use any barbells in the Regionals, so it would be a nice continuation of that theme. It's the only way I can fit in all the tests and work that I want the athletes to perform on Friday.

I'm considering Friday a peak day, and then Saturday backs off just a little in volume. Sunday will be a nice hit with some long-distance events (*run-swim-run*) and then some short, intense stuff for the final.

I hope I can get more time at Yarrow tomorrow to program and plan. I'll try to work it in. I need to have a couple of good days here before I leave for Nashville.

I'm starting to feel stressed again about running out of time. I'm considering not even going to the West Regional in Week 3 and just going to the Atlantic Regional for a day. I need to conserve my energy and really dive into the schedule to make the Games happen this year. I would hate to miss Portland because the event is at a new venue, but I think I might need do to that. Being home during Regionals would be a new thing for me. It's never happened. But our team is good, and these guys don't need me there—especially by the third week. Maybe I should stay home.

Closing down Games work for the day. CrossFit seminar work will continue through the evening once I get home.

*Tuesday, May 23, 5:08 p.m.*
I went to Yarrow a few times today for some programming sessions. While I was driving, I had an idea for an event: 21-15-9 calories on the rower or Assault bike and thrusters with a single dumbbell. Or some variant of that. The highlight of this event would not be the actual event movements but the layout. This idea actually came from the layout and then went to testing. It doesn't always work in this order. Oftentimes it's the other way around. For this one, we'd use three sets of bikes (*or rowers*) and three sets of objects to lift. This would create a true race down the floor. I really enjoy having this kind of equipment freedom at the Games. Each lane would have three rowers or bikes, but if we did this at Regionals each lane would have only one rower or bike.

I just read a post on one of the blogs that covers CrossFit, and the author referred to a Reebok post that mentioned I'm writing a book. The writer said it won't be a bestseller. That's probably very true. I also don't care. This book will be interesting to those who follow the sport closely or are really familiar with CrossFit and the CrossFit Games. This isn't for people who want to learn about CrossFit or are somewhat interested in the Games.

The reality is I'm not writing this for anybody but myself. That sounds corny, but it's the truth. I'm writing it because I want to chronicle my process of programming the Games. If I wanted to write a bestseller, I would probably just write about my time as a Navy SEAL or the life and leadership lessons I learned from 12 years in the Navy and more than a decade as Director of the CrossFit Games. That would be a bestseller because of the size of our community and my background. But I don't want to sell out like that.

I've been going through the schedule again. Due to logistics and staffing, it looks like we might need to move all the run-swim-run events to Thursday. That bums me out. I originally had the different age groups swimming on different days and the teams and individuals doing two swim events. At this stage, it's looking like that's not going to happen this year. I was also really excited about giving them their *endurance* event on Sunday, toward the end of the competition. Looks like that won't happen either. These are not changes I wanted to make, but I will make it work.

The costs and staffing demands of the original plan were prohibitive. It's much easier to do all the swimming events on one day, especially because it's an off-site event. Cost is not always a guiding factor in my decisions, but it is something I have to take into consideration. Here, I have to consider how expensive it is to run this event and how much more it would cost to conduct the run-swim-run each day from Thursday to Friday. We would have to hire the water rescue teams and the water film teams for four days instead of one.

Today I feel really behind on the programming. I feel like I should be further ahead at this stage even though I'm probably ahead of my pace in programming the other 10 editions of the Games. I just feel like I should have a lot more done.

I've decided I'm not going to Atlanta for the Regional on the third weekend. My original plan was to go to Portland and Atlanta. But now I will just go to Portland for Day 1 on the final weekend, then come home to work on the

Games stuff. It will be the first time I'll watch Regionals from home. I have great teams out there, so I'm not too worried, but it will be a little awkward for me that weekend. But it's the right decision.

*Wednesday, May 24, 3:44 p.m.*

Tomorrow I leave for the Central Regional in Nashville. Today I came into Yarrow to work on some of the schedule issues. I'm trying to figure out where to do the bike event and how to make it fit. I had to move the run-swim-run to Thursday, so I need to see what I can do with the bike event. I was originally planning on doing it Thursday. My current options are to keep it on Thursday—which makes that a very busy day—or move it to Sunday. I'm leaning toward keeping it on Thursday.

As I was going through the schedule, I thought briefly about Amanda on Thursday night. For some reason, the 9-7-5 rep scheme with heavy snatches seems like a step backward for me. They're doing 21-15-9 reps of muscle-ups and dumbbell overhead squats at Regionals, and most athletes are having little issue with it. To do a 9-7-5 at the Games seems like a step backward because of the total volume of muscle-ups. At Regionals, they're doing 45 in an event, but the total of the Games event would be only 21.

I went to my trusty pad of paper and started sketching a bunch of numerical combos down in pencil. I came up with a couple of different options. I'm looking at a 12-9-6 or maybe a 15-12-9—with the heavy barbell. Then I started thinking about maybe just a double Amanda, meaning 2 rounds of 9-7-5 reps. I like that. I wouldn't do that at 185. Maybe 155. But I would figure that out in my testing phases with a real athlete.

As I was typing this out, I thought of another possibility: 5.11 weight vests! Maybe go back to the original 9-7-5 with a vest. That's an idea I need to explore. If I want to do it, I should probably give 5.11 a heads-up. I would need 80 more vests, but they've been great about providing vests and gear, so it shouldn't be a problem.

Speaking of partners being great or not being great: In Week 1, the Assault AirBikes and AirRunners worked without any issues, so kudos to Roger for delivering a new product that worked well, and for making it happen on such short notice.

*Thursday, May 25, 10:46 p.m.*

On my flight to Nashville for the Central Regional. This is the first time the city has hosted a regional, and I'm excited to see the venue. I always enjoy seeing our new venues, what works and what doesn't work.

Tonight, I'm grabbing dinner with Dan Bailey, Rich Froning and his dad, Bill and Caity Henniger, and Karianne and Bill Anthes—and I enjoy the company of everyone in this group. I usually like doing small dinners. Karianne works for me in the Training Department, and she also helps me at some of the events on the road. At the Games, she leads the team that is assigned to work with me.

Amanda was the first workout we did when we moved from The Ranch in 2010 to the Home Depot Center *(now the StubHub Center)*. I programmed the event in memory of Amanda Miller, a 2009 CrossFit Games competitor who was diagnosed with melanoma.

*"I just competed in the CF Games less than a year ago and now I'm dying,"* she wrote on March 9, 2010.

She passed away on April 23 of that year. She was 24.

After she passed, we were still a few months from the Games, and I decided I would program a workout in memory of her. I wanted something that was like Fran but a step up in difficulty. I played with a lot of combinations but ended up with 9-7-5 reps of muscle-ups and squat snatches at 135 lb. I flipped the order with the weightlifting and gymnastics components. In Fran, the thrusters come before the pull-ups. In Amanda, I placed the gymnastics element first. At the time, I didn't consider the muscle-up an advanced skill, but it was a step above the pull-up—and that was the point. And the squat snatch at 135 lb. was obviously a step up from the thruster at 95. Understand that not many workouts back then contained squat snatches at 135, especially for reps or paired with muscle-ups. So some viewed Amanda as a heavier test, which led to its 9-7-5 rep scheme. At the time, those reps were appropriate, as was the loading.

At the 2010 CrossFit Games, Chris Spealler had the fastest time: 3:29. Games rookie Neal Maddox was second, with 3:46. Neal was judging at the 2009 Games, and he walked up to me and said, *"I will be out there one day competing with these guys."* From 2010 on, he was a regular at the CrossFit Games. He even qualified for Regionals this year but turned down the invite to focus on competing in the 35-39 Division at the CrossFit Games. Last year, when I hinted about the creation of this division, Maddox walked up to me at an event and told me he would win it. I love Neal's attitude and confidence. He always goes into the competition with the mindset that he can win. Chris Spealler also qualified for the Games in the 35-39 Division this year. That actually surprised me, and I'm proud of him.

In 2010, a new unknown kid from Tennessee had the third fastest Amanda time: 3:47. He would go on to take second overall, and he eventually dominated the sport. That was Rich Froning, of course.

Another future champ, Ben Smith, had the fifth fastest time: 4:01. In 2017, Smith did Amanda at 185 lb. in 4:06, and Josh Bridges recently posted a video in which he does it with the same load in 3:36. His time was 10 seconds better than our second-fastest time at 135 in 2010. That's how far the sport has progressed.

On the female side of the 2010 Games, Kristan Clever had the fastest time, with 5:04. The next female to finish the event was almost two full minutes behind, at 7:02. That was Camille Leblanc-Bazinet, an unknown from Canada. She would go on to win the CrossFit Games in 2014 and become one of the most liked and popular athletes in our sport. Last week, she qualified for the CrossFit Games again.

At this stage, I plan on having Amanda as the first test in the Coliseum in Madison, just as it was the first event in the stadium in Carson. It won't be the first event overall, but it will be the first CrossFit event once we're done with Thursday's outdoor tests.

My challenge now is finding the right variant of Amanda. I don't want to do the original version, but I want to do something similar. Two rounds is not a bad idea, but it's very similar to Double DT, which we recently did at the Games. That's a turnoff in my mind. Another option is just adding a round on each end, something like this: 11-9-7-5-3 reps. And I'd keep the weight at 135. I actually hate that the default method of making a workout or test harder is always increasing the weight. It doesn't have to be like that. I like the idea of 11-9-7-5-3 reps at 135 lb. I think that could still be very fast and very hard. It would be 35 total reps of muscle-ups and squat snatches at 135. In Event 5 of the 2017 Regionals, athletes are doing 45 muscle-ups in a couplet, and the fastest times are about 6 minutes. I also actually really like the 5-round format of 11-9-7-5-3. Typically, you see declining rep counts in

3-round workouts. Rarely do you see 5 rounds. I might start testing this with athletes as early as next week, and I can't wait. This will be the first pure CrossFit event I'll test for the 2017 CrossFit Games. Now I'm getting excited.

Creating the schedule for the Games is very challenging this year. Before I just created a schedule for teams and individuals, and that alone is pretty hard, but now I have multiple venues with multiple divisions, so it's exponentially harder. I'm close to having a schedule I will work off, and I can't wait to start really planning and testing actual events. That's why it's exciting to think about Amanda and the effects of its possible variants.

I'm thinking about Amanda's layout. If we do 3 rounds, I would want 3 sets of rings spread across the floor. That way athletes never walk backward and always move forward. It would take a ton of gear, but it would look great—and it would also mean three sets of barbells. If we did the 5-round version, it would require five rigs. Bill might not be excited about that, but it would be an epic sight on the floor. I need to see if it will fit.

Speaking of floor plans, Justin and J-Mac had a good idea to create lane-number markers to place on the floor at Regionals. They will be placed in different locations depending on the event. Instead of having to follow the lane back to the rig to determine which one it is, you can just see the number on the floor. It's a really good idea and something we are putting in play this weekend at the two North American competitions. I'm not sure if we'll be able to pull it off for Australia because we likely don't have time to get the necessary materials down there.

*Friday, May 26, 7:41 p.m.*
Day 1 at the Central Regional. The venue is a convention center. The space is very nice and large. Convention centers have the benefit of being a blank canvas, and we come in and create exactly what we need for the event. As long as we build the right layout, convention centers usually make great venues. This layout was nice, and the venue was clean and seemed new.

One big miss: The bleachers are low. They are not any lower than most bleachers we use, but if you are sitting in rows one to four or so, it's hard to see the floor. I spoke with J-Mac about this, and he said we could put them on risers to correct that problem. But that would be a significant cost increase. If the bleachers we had today were on risers, the event and venue would have been next level. As it is, it's still a great venue and a great setup.

A ton of people showed up on Friday. Saturday is going to be crazy, I imagine, but I'm currently flying to the California Regional, where I will spend Saturday and Sunday.

My mind isn't really on Regionals right now, though. I'm still doing what I need to do and seeing what I need to see, but I'm consumed by Games planning. I actually wish I wasn't traveling to any of the Regionals so I could work on the Games. Luckily, I'm making progress on the Games, and I had a couple of good discussions today with some key people.

I spoke to Bill about the Worms. Currently, the Worms have heavy sections in the front (*80 lb. for men and 60 lb. for women*), medium sections in the middle (*70/55 lb.*), and light sections in the back (*60/50 lb.*). When I was in California, I saw the unpacked Worms and realized they ship the bags out of the Worms and then assemble them at each location. *"Why not just make Worms from the heavy, medium or light bags?"* I thought. For example, we could take only the heavy men's and women's sections and put them in the Worm so the sections are 80/60/80/60/80/60 lb. Then we could do the same thing to make Worms with sections of only 70/55 lb. and 60/50 lb. With this plan, we would have four Worms: the current Worm, plus light, medium and heavy variations (*the medium variation would actually weigh the same as the current Worm, but the loading would be different*).

Man, it will be so cool to be able to introduce new Worm weights at the Games, and then eventually carry that over to Regionals. Honestly, I don't know why it's taken so long for us to come up with this idea. I discussed it with Bill, and he loved it. I actually talked to him about making the shells different colors. If he can pull that off, it would be great.

I also sat down with Danny Rodgers and J-Mac in a private room and discussed the bike event. I let J-Mac create the course. On paper, it looks like he did a great job with the format of the event and the course. Start to finish, the event will take around three hours on Thursday. We have two heats of 20 people for each gender, and they'll race three or four laps around the course.

As we discussed it, I realized there is the potential for some really great riders to be in both heats. I want all the great riders to be in one heat together, so I suggested time trials to seed them. That way the bottom 20 athletes from the time trials would race together, and the top 20 athletes would race in another heat. This will create a much better competition.

Johnny quickly put together a plan and sent it to me. Time trials will have to happen on Tuesday or Wednesday, but I am OK with that.

I brought up one question we left unanswered at this point: If we would limit an athlete's potential final placing based on the time trial. For example, if I finished the time trial with a time that left me in 30th place, I would be in the 21-40 heat, not the main-event heat with the top qualifiers. In this scenario, though, athletes from the lower heat might log times faster than those in the premier heat. The question is if riders in the bottom heat will compete only for placings from 21 to 40 or if they can place higher by logging times faster than those of the athletes in the top heat. In this scenario, the fastest time could come from what was supposed to be the slower heat. Johnny suggested one option I didn't like at the time: We could score the time trials for points. Thinking back, that's actually not a bad idea. But I said we'd come back to this detail and discuss the event at length later. For now, I'm very happy with the format, and I think we should go forward.

Last night I went to bed thinking that I don't want to wake up to a rash of injuries from the Pacific Regional because of Individual Event 2. I woke up at 5. I couldn't really sleep, and 5 is early for me. I normally wake up at 6. I checked my phone immediately to see what the team from Australia had reported to me, and it looked like there were three injuries on Event 2. Damn, that sucks.

When I looked closer at the emails I had been sent, it looked like two athletes had withdrawn prior to the start of the event, and we had one injury actually happen on the floor.

A few hours later, I closely watched the Central individuals in Event 2. Everyone was fine in Heat 1. I actually found myself surprised that injuries are happening at all. It seems crazy to me. It isn't asking that much of them, and even the fast guys on this event are not that fast, meaning their movement doesn't appear completely reckless.

In the second heat, one athlete looked like he was having issues. I had Chuck Carswell talk to him, and turns out the athlete had sustained an injury prior to the competition, not during. In the next heat, Nick Urankar didn't meet the minimum work requirement and pulled out of the competition. He basically walked onto the floor and didn't do a single rep. He said he had also injured himself in training.

In the final heat, it looked like nobody was injured. As I was leaving the venue, I congratulated Dan Bailey on how well he did, and he pulled me aside and told me he thought he tore something on the set of 21. Damn, that sucks. He still managed to post a very fast time and took second overall.

I hate to see people get injured, especially when they are good friends of mine. That makes it even worse.

At the airport, I watched the California Regional stream closely, and I saw Henry Lopez sustain an injury. I think he was the only one. Later in the evening, Sam Dancer posted a pic and said he had sustained an injury in training. We are still seeing injuries from this event, though not as many in a single Regional. But we are also seeing some amazing performances, and an overwhelming majority of the competitors have no issues.

I enjoyed seeing a bunch of people I like and consider good friends, such as Rich Froning, Dan Bailey, Julie Foucher and Brooke Wells. I have known Rich for seven years and consider us close. We keep in regular contact, we find it easy to relate to each other, and we share common interests. I hung out with him and his team, and I met his new baby. I called him Rich Jr. Jr. The child was so small. It's been a long time since I've seen a baby. I'm really glad the baby phase of my life is over. I can't imagine doing that again. Rich, of course, dominated the competition with his team. He told me Event 2 really hurt, and that made me happy. It's not often Rich gives feedback like that, so I will take it when I can.

I had dinner with Dan last night and hung out with him a little today. He didn't do great on Event 1 but had a very fast time on Event 2 to take second. But it looks like he's injured. I really hope it's not as bad as he thinks and he can get through the weekend and back to the Games.

Tonight at the airport, I texted him and asked how the injury was. He said it still hurt.

Of all the athletes, Dan is one of the ones I accidentally grew close to. We kind of grew to be good friends. I think it all started when we did CrossFit's Big Sky excursion. One year, it was about two weeks after the Games. I didn't want to do it, but it's an obligation due to my role in CrossFit. I drove my Ranger Rover Sport—which is all kitted out for off-road excursions—from the Bay Area to Big Sky, Montana, solo. It was a great drive. I got to clear my head and see a lot of great American landscape I had never seen before.

The original plan was to follow Pat Sherwood, Erik Preston, Ian Wittenber and Tyson Oldroyd, who were riding motorcycles to Big Sky. But early on we got separated, and I never rejoined them.

Big Sky was fun—lots of hiking, lots of drinking, lots of socializing and hanging out with affiliate owners. Once the trip was over, I was looking at a return drive to California. Dan and I knew each other through work trips like this but were not close friends. I knew he was easygoing and didn't have many attachments, so I walked up to him and said, "*Hey, Dan. You're going to ride back with me to Santa Cruz*." He said, "*OK.*"

The next morning, not really knowing each other that well, we got in the truck together and started an epic drive back. We spoke a lot about religion—he did most of the talking—and his life. We stopped in Reno, spent the night and then barreled home the next day. He never drove once. He also lost one of his bags on the trip. I think he left it in Big Sky. He swears up and down that he left it in my truck and I just threw it away. I like that version of the story, but it's not true. I wouldn't do that to him.

Julie and I also go back a few years because she's been a competitor for so long. Often, I end up becoming friends with athletes because of the amount of time we spend together at the Games, at Regionals, at the Invitational and at special events we invite them to attend. In Julie's case *(and Rich's)*, she became a member of CrossFit's Level 1 Seminar Staff. Julie works a seminar a month or so and loves teaching in that environment. She does a great job. She competed on a team at the Regional, and we didn't get to catch up. But we said hi to each other.

Brooke Wells has been to the Games for the previous two years, but I really didn't get to know her there. I did have a little exchange with her after one of the Games because her mom sent me a DM saying how nice I was and thanked me for treating her daughter well. I told Brooke, and she said she knew about it and was embarrassed.

Brooke was on the Invitational team that competed in Toronto, Canada, in November 2016. That's where I really got to know her and spend time with her, and we invited her to compete in Mexico City as part of the announcement of Open Workout 17.4.

I spoke to her today before the event started, and she was in a good head space. She came out very hot on Event 1 and was in second for three or four rounds but then quickly fell off. Afterward, I saw her in the warm-up area, and she didn't look happy at all. I offered a couple of words of encouragement and left her and Ben Bergeron, her coach, to do their thing. She later did great in Event 2, and when I saw her afterward she said she felt better and thought she overheated during Event 1.

The crowd was great. I posed for lots of photos with people, and a common theme I'm seeing across all Regionals is the *"Dave Castro is a prick"* shirts. That T-shirt seems to have done well for the Good Dudes guys.

*(Something very funny just happened to me on this flight: As I was typing that story above, a flight attendant came up to me and said, "I have to say I am really sorry I don't have my 'Dave Castro is a prick' T-shirt right now." She went on to talk about where she does CrossFit and said she is a big fan. I like meeting CrossFit people around the world.)*

I'm happy to be heading back home for the next two days of Regionals. I'll be able to get some work done on the Games. We have family in town this weekend, so I imagine I'll spend my day at the Regional and then go to Yarrow to do some programming. For me, having family in town means the kids are occupied and I can spend more time doing work.

It's 12:41 a.m. Central time. I've been traveling for the last six hours, and I'm 35 minutes away from landing in San Diego. I figured I would talk a little bit about what I saw at the California Regional today via the stream.

I'm not surprised Christian Lucero is doing so well. He was strong at the Regional in 2016 and made a great showing at the Games last year. More importantly, he has a hunger and a fighting spirit that is often missing from a lot of other top competitors. Josh Bridges also has hunger, and he's doing great, as expected. We'll see how the heavy kettlebells and sandbags treat him. He practices those things a lot, and he's good at them, but the guys who are 20-40 lb. heavier and also very fit have an advantage over him through body size alone. But his heart is huge, and that counts for a lot. I was really surprised to see Garret Fisher do so well on Event 1. Then he didn't do so well on Event 2. I hope he didn't hurt himself.

On the female side, it doesn't seem like there are any dominant players. Common names, yes, but no clear-cut favorite. I feel like there was a brief phase when Lauren Fisher was a dominant athlete at these events, but it seems like that has passed. She's still great, but she's not cleaning house like she did in her first two years on the scene.

Val Voboril is doing great. That's a big surprise to me. I hope she continues to do well, but I don't know if she will. I honestly don't think so—but I really want her to succeed.

Becca Voigt looks good, too, but she needs a few more strong events to qualify for the Games. I saw Lindsey Valenzuela's face when she finished Event 2, and it was not happy. She is not doing well, and her face showed as much when she crossed the line. It looks like she has no shot at making it this year. I imagine she'll make another run next year, hopefully a good comeback.

Tomorrow, I'll reverse the pattern and watch the Central Regional on my iPad while watching the California Regional in person.

*Sunday, May 28, 6:56 p.m.*
Wow, what a competition. California always has drama and intrigue.

I just got home from the event and had dinner, and I'm still processing everything. I think I'll start by addressing the Christian Lucero *"injury."*

Lucero was crushing the competition. He took second in Event 1 and first in Event 2, the snatch/ring-dip event. On Saturday, he was almost as impressive, and he finished the afternoon in solid first-place position over Josh Bridges. At one point, I walked up and congratulated Christian and told him how proud I was of how he was doing. I told him I liked his approach to training and competing and appreciated how he was always trying to win. Everything was going great.

Later, he asked if we could talk at the end of the day Saturday. I told him we could. I later found him alone by the ice buckets and asked him what he wanted to discuss. He said he had been getting his testosterone levels checked on a weekly basis because his levels were really low after the 2016 Games. Every week he gets them checked, and they have been fine—except last week. The week before Regionals started, he had his levels tested, and they were very high, so he's concerned he might not pass a test that would be mandatory here. So he might pull out of Day 3 because he doesn't want to pop positive and make the sport look bad.

I was very surprised by all of this. Frankly, I didn't want to hear it. Lots of red flags were going up in my mind.

I said, *"Hey, here is the deal: You need to talk to my guy who is in charge of the testing program and explain what you have going on."* It all sounded very suspicious, and I didn't want to give him the wrong guidance or put us in an awkward position, so the best thing I could do was tell him to talk to Stephane Rochet, who is in charge of our drug-testing protocol.

Lucero talked to Stephane that evening, and Stephane called me Saturday night. He explained what Lucero had told him and said it's a very unique situation—to put it lightly. I asked him where the situation is at now, and he said that Lucero will decide tomorrow if he will continue or withdraw. No matter what he does, the situation is very unique and suspicious. Stephane suggested we test Lucero regardless. We have the right, and, frankly, the obligation, to test any athlete in the field, especially if there are suspicious circumstances. At this stage, we decided to leave the issue to the next day and see what Lucero decides to do.

Sunday rolls around, and I see Christian warming up. In my mind, I am like, *"OK, cool. He's going to go through the comp and do the test and see what happens."* At this point I think he must be innocent, and it's all a mistake.

Well, Event 5 starts, and I don't see if he attempts a rep or not, but within minutes he's standing on the floor doing zero work and holding his chest. He's making it seem like he has a pec injury. I see him doing that on the floor, and I think, *"What bullshit."* He decided to take a route I didn't even expect or anticipate. He decided to take the floor and basically fake an injury—fake an injury to a body part that's been prone to injury. But let's not forget he took first on Event 2, the ring-dip event, and then continued on Day 2 and did great. But then on Day 3 he has a pec injury that pops up on Event 5, the muscle-up event in which nobody else injured themselves at Regionals. I was furious.

Our event director and team took him off the floor and brought him to the back area once his heat was over. He refused any medical assessment or treatment from our docs. He said his own guy would check him out, but he absolutely didn't want our team to check him. He and his coach asked if he could just leave, but we said no. The team then let him know that he was going to be tested. That was news he was not expecting. Again, we have the right to test any member of the field at any time. Our team took a sample from him, and then he was released to do his own thing.

I am very surprised at how this played out, and frankly I'm really disappointed in how he handled it. We'll have the test results back in a few weeks, and I'll be very surprised if he doesn't test positive for something. If he does, we'll have to announce the results, and this will for sure be one of the biggest stories of this season.

I actually like Christian and was hoping he would make it to the Games and excel, but now I am questioning his character and his actions. I could be wrong, and he could be completely clean. Time will tell.

The female competition was fun. I was very happy Chyna Cho won, and I can't believe Val Voboril will be back in the Individual competition at the Games after a two-year hiatus. Val had already qualified for the Masters competition in the 35-39 Division, and after Day 2 I discussed what her choice would be if she qualified in the Individual division, too. She said Individual for sure. She told me it's a higher honor, and there won't always be Individual competition in her future—but there will always be the possibility of Masters competition.

Rebecca Voigt missed qualifying. It would have been her 10th year in a row. It was sad but not totally unexpected. New people come up, and athletes lose a step once age starts creeping up. Becca has been on the scene for a decade, and her streak of Individual Games qualification is over, but she also qualified for the Masters competition and can still compete there.

One last dramatic, positive thing happened this wild weekend: Earlier in the competition, Julian Alcaraz mentioned to someone on our media team that he was thinking about giving up his Games spot—should he qualify—because he has a baby due in August during or around the Games. I found this out on Saturday, so I spoke to Julian about it, and he had become very solid on giving up the spot. I said I would ask him again tomorrow just to be sure.

Julian finished fourth overall, so I briefed our production team, Boz and Josh Gallegos, who was our floor MC. First, I would walk onto the floor and ask Julian to confirm his decision to give up the spot. I did that once Event 6 was over. Second, the team would then announce the five athletes who had qualified for the Games. Third, Josh would then dramatically announce that

Julian had given up his spot to be with his family, so we would award his spot to the sixth-place finisher. That's how it played out, and it was dramatic.

I admire Julian for his decision. I wish he were competing, but now he will be a great guy to test workouts for me because he lives in Orange County, California, about 45 minutes away from Yarrow. I used him sparingly in that role last year. This year, I think I'll use him on a more regular basis. I talked to him about that after the event, and he said he would be honored to help me test. I said, "*Stay ready and expect a call from me soon.*"

This Regional was unique. Because of what happened with Christian and Julian, we essentially have the sixth- and seventh-place finishers going to the Games. Under normal circumstances, they would not have made it. But it's the California Regional, so of course there is drama.

Two more notes before I take the rest of the evening off.

First, I thought I would be able to go to the competition and then do Games programming in the evening, but I wasn't able to do that on either evening. I'm disappointed, but I'm excited about diving in hard this week and only having one Regional to attend.

Second, Nick Urankar had an injured pec that didn't allow him to finish Event 2 at the Central Regional. I don't think Nick did any dips at all in the event. I felt bad for the guy. I hate the injuries in this year's competition. Well, today someone sends me a video of Nick in the USAW area of our Regional event, and he's lifting weights in front of a large crowd. He PRs his snatch at over 300 lb.

This guy pulls out of the competition for a pec injury but two days later PRs his snatch. I texted Dan and asked him if he could snatch right now. He said he is in too much pain to take a 45-lb. barbell overhead.

The team then suggests to me that we should test Urankar. We have that right, and I said, "*Let's do it.*" So they called him up and said he needed to come back to the venue to be tested.

*Monday, May 29, 8:51 p.m.*
I had a couple of good sessions at Yarrow today—not too long. It's Memorial Day, and I'm getting some much-needed rest. I looked over the schedule again, and I feel it's becoming firm. I also sent Pat an email so we can get on another call and go over the Age Group schedules.

I also had a couple of other thoughts.

I'm having the Games athletes do Amanda—or some variant—on Thursday, then possibly a squat-snatch test on Friday. I was thinking clean and jerk on Saturday, but that's a ton of squatting three days in a row, and we haven't even included thrusters in there yet. They'll probably come Sunday. So that pushes me in the direction of possibly making Saturday's clean and jerk either a power clean and jerk or just a power clean. A power-clean speed ladder would be a very exciting event.

A few days ago, I thought about bringing the Banger back. The Banger was that big piece of steel we had athletes hammer down the floor with a sledgehammer in various ways at the 2012 Games. I asked Bill if he could send me one, and he said he would have to find a Banger. I know we have one in the Scotts Valley office. It's currently a prop on the Update Show. I told Bill that I would just have that one delivered, and I was wondering who could make the drive, which is seven or eight hours.

Greg was in town for Regionals, and I found out he was flying up to Northern California in our plane. I texted Michael Buttenob, our pilot, and asked him what time he would be in Watsonville, the airport we fly into. He said around 2 p.m., so I contacted the team at the office and had someone take the Banger to the plane. They loaded it in, and Mike flew it back down to Carlsbad. I met him at the airport at 5, and it took four people to unload it and put it in the back of my truck. I'm excited about having the Banger and testing some potential events with it. It might be a nice addition to the 2017 Games.

*Tuesday, May 30, 7:34 p.m.*
I had a few good sessions planning and programming at Yarrow. During the first session, I focused on some event stuff and played around with ideas for a Team workout and the Individual workout that might have burpees over a wall. I thought of a few other ways of doing that event. I might have them do burpees over the Pig, a big implement we used in 2015 at the Games. I even had a crazy idea of using hay bales. I asked Bill how many Pigs he has left, and he said only eight, so if we need more, he needs to know now. I don't think we will use them. They're very large and costly to build.

The original barricades I had Bill send me won't work either because they are cost prohibitive in the quantities I want. Maybe hay bales would work just fine. Actually, maybe we could use the hay bales to mark the bike course and then repurpose them for this event. The original plan was to have the athletes do a burpee and clean an object over the wall, then climb over the wall. One issue I'm running into now as the Games slowly come together: We already have so much cleaning or clean-like movements. I'm not yet at the point where I compare all the movements I've programmed, but at a glance I can see a lot of big hip-opening movements in what I have planned. Amanda's snatches, snatches for load, a speed clean ladder, a burpee over a wall with a clean—a lot of hip-opening movements.

Most of these thoughts occurred during my morning session.

This afternoon, I came in and had a good couple of hours diving into the schedule and really making some great changes to the plan and flow of the overall show. When working on the schedule, I'm thinking a lot about the fan experience and how they will or will not enjoy the show.

Today I got a good grasp of Thursday, but that means an 8-a.m. start, and we end around 6:30 p.m. I don't want Day 1 to be really late. Late days usually fall on the second or third day of competition.

I also made some good progress on Friday's schedule. Friday will essentially be a loaded day because I have the individuals doing four events. I figured out where and how things would go with the three Team events that day. To make it work, I have to use 20-person heats in both Individual CrossFit tests in the Coliseum. That will give me the time I need—and I dropped one event time to 15 from 20 minutes.

I also made a lot of progress on Saturday and came up with a good flow. I've pretty much decided the Saturday lift will be a power-clean speed ladder. In years past, athletes advanced to different stages, but this clean ladder will be like the one we did at Regionals last year: one time through an ascending ladder, with time caps at lower weights. I also might add a small secondary component to it, like a row or Assault bike, or maybe even some sort of gymnastics movement. Or maybe double-unders. I don't know. I have to play this one out on paper some more. But I made a big addition to this plan: I'm going to have the teams do this event, too.

Playing with the schedule tonight basically made me decide on something like this: We build the floor for Individual female competitors. Because it's a speed clean ladder, we will have a lot of bars on the floor—possibly six to eight per lane, multiplied by 10 lanes. We could run four heats of Team women through a variant of the test. The floor stays the same, and four heats of Individual women go through. We have a big break to switch to male weights and then run through four heats of Team men. Then we have four heats of male Individual athletes go through the same bars. This is one way of doing it.

I felt good today. It was great to spend so much time at Yarrow getting some of this work done. At one point, I kind of thought that maybe I should also go to the Regional in Atlanta this weekend, but then I snapped out of it and realized it will be better to stay home and get a ton of work done for the Games.

*Wednesday, May 31, 6:59 p.m.*

Today was more scheduling. I accomplished a lot on it. I think it's close to being set. Now I just need to program the actual blocks and exactly what happens in them. That sounds more dramatic than it is, and a lot of stuff is already programmed. All of Thursday is programmed—kinda. Run-Swim-Run, bike, Amanda *(I just need to figure out what variant)*. Some of Friday is done: O-course, snatch, two CrossFit events *(both of which need to be programmed)*. Saturday: one north-lot run workout, speed power-clean ladder and a CrossFit event. Sunday: work event and CrossFit event or events.

In terms of Thursday and Friday, the schedule is tight and set. For Saturday and Sunday, I have some wiggle room. As of now, I have Saturday ending around 8, so that gives me room to flex. I can make heats longer or even add an event.

I also had a call with Pat today about the Masters schedule. I had to move a lot of things around for the individuals, and because I placed all the Run-Swim-Run events on the same day, it changed his schedule, too. We talked through all the age divisions, where everything is and what I expect for each. We didn't go over workouts but themes for what type of workout would work in which venue or area.

Also talked to Justin today about our upcoming June meeting. That's where I'll brief all the workouts to our small team. I laughed and said, *"Well, I will have 60-70 percent of it done. Not all of it."*

That meeting is in about 26 days, so I have time to get a lot done.

I reached out to Julian and scheduled a time for him to test events this weekend. He said he is not a good swimmer or basketball player because he is brown.

*"Don't worry,"* I said. *"You won't have to test those things."*

I'm going to have him test a variant of the new Amanda I want to do—probably a 5-round version. I'm excited about that.

## JUNE 2017

*Thursday, June 1, 12:53 p.m.*

I came into Yarrow a couple of hours ago, and I've had a great planning session. I leave for Portland and the West Regional in a few hours, so this was a good push forward. I feel like I made progress on a couple of events. Even if it wasn't a lot, I made some progress, which makes me feel good.

The first thing I had to take care of was figuring out what I'm going to have Julian Alcaraz test. I have him set up to test with me on Saturday.

We extended our competition floor in Madison to 130 feet and are able to put five rigs on there for muscle-ups. It will look epic in scale. Because we can fit five rigs, I'm planning and programming around a 5-round variant of Amanda. One of my first thoughts was double Amanda, or heavy Amanda, but we've done Double DT and Heavy DT in previous years. So I'm leaning toward extending Amanda. One version is 11-9-7-5-3, for 35 reps of each movement. Another version is 13-11-9-7-5, for 45 reps of each movement. I like that version because the ring totals are low in each round to entice people to go unbroken. The total work is 45 reps, which they did at Regionals, but these will be very different tests. This one will be more chaotic and rushed. We'll lay this out on the floor in one continuous race, which will look great.

So on Saturday Julian tests 11-9-7-5-3. As of right now, I have an 11-minute time cap and 15-minute heats. Guys do the regular version in 3 minutes, so I think this version should take around 6-8 minutes, maybe even high fives for the fastest.

I had an interesting idea I sent to Bill. It might not work, but I want to experiment with taking a normal round bumper plate and making one side flat. In theory, you can set the bar down on the flat side, and it won't roll around on the competition floor. But in typing this out, it might be hard to impossible to have the flat sides of both plates line up. Either way, Bill said he will work on a set to send me. This is not for this year's Games, just for testing. Maybe one day we use it, or it might just end up being a bad idea. But we'll find out.

I'm pretty set on Friday night closing with some sort of Banger finale. Assault bike 30 calories or so and drive the Banger down the floor 50 feet. I'm going to get that tested in the next few weeks.

I started playing with another Friday event. This one needs to allow heats of 20, so that means no barbells and not a lot of room. I pulled out two GHDs and put them side by side to see how much room I would have. I can make it fit, so I sketched out a 3-round event of X *(high)* GHD reps, X *(lower)* deadlifts—maybe again with kettlebells—and finally maybe a SkiErg. As I was playing this out and thinking about all the pulling going on already, I wondered what else would play well here. A push press would complement the GHD and SkiErg nicely and give a break from the pulling-heavy theme that's creeping in. A single-arm heavy-ish push press with a dumbbell would be great. I like that idea. If Julian is feeling good on Saturday, maybe I'll have him test that event. At this stage, the plan is probably going to change dramatically.

I was making such good progress on Saturday that I decided to take a look at Sunday. As of now, my *"chaos"* event has not found a place in the schedule. And my Sunday schedule has two events. Looking hard at everything the athletes will have done at that point and comparing the volume to what we have done in years past on Sunday, I decided to add a third event on Sunday. I think I can make a great show of this. I texted Justin and asked him what time he wants to end Sunday, and he said it's up to us. So I asked him what he preferred. He said 5 or 6 p.m. So I currently have Sunday ending at 6:05.

OK. Leaving Yarrow so I can get ready to head to the airport to go to Portland for my final Regional event of 2017. I'm feeling really good about where I am with the Games and how everything is moving forward.

*5:22 p.m.*
I'm on my flight to Portland. This is a two-hour flight, and much easier than most of my travel of late. The last two weekends of flights to four Regionals all required multiple connections. It seemed to take forever. This flight is direct and two hours—a nice change from the epically long travel days. My whole adult life has been spent in careers that require me to travel, and I travel a lot. I really don't enjoy it anymore. I don't like to travel for fun or to see new places. At this stage, I like to stay home or drive or ride places, but the idea of getting on a plane for fun does not appeal to me anymore.

I have a few sewing projects I'm working on that need to be finished, but right now sewing has taken a back seat in my life. Sewing is an interesting hobby of mine, and most people are surprised that I do it. I think in the last year it has really picked up. Before that, my sewing was sparse.

I learned how to sew almost 20 years ago. When I enlisted in the Navy at the young age of 19, I had to choose a vocation. In the Navy, it's called an "A" school. The point of this school was to learn a job in the regular Navy. That was needed because I really wanted to be a Navy SEAL, which was very unlikely, at least according to my recruiters and the statistics. So when they gave me a choice of vocations, I selected parachute rigger. It sounded cool to me. I would get to learn how to pack parachutes, and I thought it would help me accomplish my goal of becoming a SEAL.

I went to boot camp in February 1997 and spent two months in the cold town of Great Lakes, Illinois. I had never been exposed to such cold temperatures growing up in the Monterey Bay area. After boot camp, I came home for a few weeks' leave, at which point I found out that my girlfriend when I went to boot camp had left me for a friend of mine. Then I went out to Pensacola, Florida, where the A school was located. That was another two months. I spent most of my time focused on training for BUD/S. I also found out the parachute rigging I was going to learn wasn't for skydivers like I imagined but for ejection seats in Naval aircraft. We learned how to repair and maintain all types of rescue gear used in aviation, and we learned how to sew. I had never sewn in my life, but I took an interest in it and enjoyed it. The first thing we made was a canvas tool bag I have to this day. Over the years, I sewed patches on it from all the SEAL teams I was stationed at.

After graduating A school, I eventually went to BUD/S and made it through in one push. Once at a SEAL team, I quickly learned how valuable my sewing skills were. I sewed and modified a lot of gear for myself and others. I actually became pretty good at it. I bought my first industrial-strength sewing machine from a teammate for $1,000 in early 2000. That machine followed me around to the various places I lived while in Virginia Beach, Virginia. In 2007, when I was stationed in Monterey for the Defense Language Institute (DLI), I put the sewing machine in our shop at The Ranch. From the DLI I was transferred to Coronado to be a BUD/S instructor. I moved with my family—one daughter at the time—to a small house in San Diego. The house was only 1,200 square feet, so I decided to leave the sewing machine at The Ranch. It takes up a ton of room, and I figured I was past that stage.

I eventually got the itch to continue sewing, so I started researching industrial-strength home machines. The market is tiny. Most industrial sewing machines come with a big table and take up tons of room. I eventually came across a company called Sailrite, which makes a great portable industrial-strength sewing machine. I purchased one, and it became a workhorse for me when I felt like sewing. The only problem was that whenever I wanted to sew, I would have to pull everything out, set it up and then put everything away. This was how I would sew from about 2007 until last year. I sewed very infrequently, but I had the capacity when I wanted to make something. A couple of years ago, I was asking Bill about sewing leathers and how his company does it. Seeing my interest, he sent me a great leather hand sewing machine and some leather to work with. I was so intimidated by the thought of trying to learn how to sew with leather and that machine. It probably sat unopened in my garage for two years.

In late November or December 2016, I had already been in Yarrow for most of the year, and I realized I had a lot of room. I decided to move my small Sailrite machine and the machine Bill gave me over to the office. I set them both up and started sewing, sewing and sewing some more. Through a good friend of mine who was in the Navy with me and is now on our Seminar Staff, I was able to track down the original pattern for my tool bag that I made almost 20 years ago. So I made a bunch of those. I made one for each of my two girls and my wife. I also made one for Bill. I learned how to sew a dopp kit, which isn't hard, and I've since made a bunch of those, too. In this process, I started dabbling with waxed canvas and leather. Previously, I usually only worked with Cordura nylons.

I eventually hauled my first sewing machine from The Ranch down to the Yarrow office, so my sewing-machine fleet grew to three. That machine needed some repairs, so I had a local guy come over and work on it. He told me I needed a different type of machine for what I was doing, something even more heavy duty. I ignored him. A few months later, I had more machine issues, and I had him come over to make repairs. He told me I needed a heavier machine. I didn't ignore him the second time. He helped me find a used one for $1,000, and I bought it. Now my fleet of sewing machines is at four. I want a fifth machine, but I'll probably wait until after the Games to purchase it.

I still sew sometimes to step away from work stuff, and it makes for a good break. It's a hobby I really enjoy, and I hope to keep improving. I enjoy making gifts for people but don't know if I'll ever make anything for retail. People have suggested I should, and I imagine if I made some small-batch items they would do OK. Since I have the machines, I've sometimes thought I might as well put them to work by hiring someone to make stuff for me that I could sell. I don't know right now. At this point, that's all distraction from what I should be doing: programming the Games.

*Friday, June 2, 7:11 p.m.*

I'm currently flying back to San Diego from the West Regional. It was a great setup, much better than last year at the Moda Center. The Moda Center is the home of the NBA's Portland Trail Blazers, and the stadium was way too big for the West Regional and its fans. We had lots of empty seats. This year, we were at a convention center, and it gave us the ability to set up the bleachers and the layout to our exact needs. The spectator demand at this Regional is generally not as high, and the convention center allows us to have really large warm-up and athlete areas, plus a great volunteer area.

While I was at the event, I set up my computer and iPad to watch the Event 2 heats from Madrid and Atlanta. It appeared two people were hurt in Europe, one before and one during the event. On the live stream from the Atlantic Regional, I saw Jeff Evans stop on the event. From what I'm being told, he came in with the injury. I saw another athlete stop, too.

In Portland, Ben Stoneberg stopped in the middle of the event because he was tweaked going into the weekend and didn't want to do more damage. I respect that decision—self-preservation for long-term training.

I don't know the final tally, but I know I'm not happy with the number of injuries. There has been lots of speculation as to why they happened. I've heard lots of good reasons and some poor explanations. I don't think it was the programming. I believe that and will continue to believe it—not just because I programmed the event but largely because so many people had no issue with it. Yes, the injury percentage was high, but an overwhelming majority were fine. I spoke a little about this today when I was on the show with the crew. One of the points I addressed was the fact that I don't like how people are not addressing the different degrees of injury severity. Not everyone is *"tearing a pec,"* which insinuates a complete tear of the pectoral muscle from the humerus. A small number of athletes have a complete tear, and others have partial tears or strains. There are varying degrees of severity.

Will I program ring dips again? Yes, of course. The ring dip is a basic CrossFit movement. Ring dips are not irresponsible or reckless. Will they be programmed in the same workout or the same rep scheme? I'm not sure yet. Time will tell.

I watched Event 1 of the Atlantic men's competition on the stream, and I was really surprised at how slow Ben Smith started. His squats were slow and deliberate. There is a time for that, but it's not an appropriate strategy at the beginning of Event 1. Ben ended up finishing in 18th place—not a great showing. Noah Ohlsen, on the other hand, had a great race with Jacob Anderson, who was directly next to him. Anderson was leading most of the way until the last few rounds, when Noah made a push and passed him to take the event win.

In Event 2, Ben finished 19th. At the end of the day, he was tied for 19th overall (100 points) with a handful of other guys. Dave Eubanks, our scoring lead, was in Portland with me and said that Ben basically doesn't have a chance. I'm surprised by that, so I had my team check in with him to find out what's wrong. Maybe he's injured, too. The report came back that he is not injured but might be slowly recovering from doing Murph on Monday. If that's true, it would be unfortunate. I would not advise an athlete to do Murph a few days before a Regional. Save it for after the event, not a few days before.

On the men's side in Portland, Cody Anderson had a great Day 1. I think he'll slide back a little on Day 2, which doesn't really favor little guys. I also think he'll have a hard time getting back to the Games, but he set himself up in a great position to make a legit run. Cole Sager had a solid day and is sitting in seventh. Brent Fikowski had a great day and is in the top five. I had a short yet pleasant conversation with him before I left the venue. He's an interesting guy, but I like him.

On the women's side of the West Regional, Tia Wright, who has missed out on the Games multiple times, had a great start and beat Carleen Mathews toward the very end of Event 1. After one day, Carleen holds the overall lead. Surprisingly, Emily Abbott is not sitting in the top five after Day 1. During Event 2, Emily's judge was very loose on her air squats, and I actually had the head judge go watch her because she was not opening up at the top. I saw her on the way out and mentioned that to her. She didn't appreciate it and snapped back at me that she was meeting the standard. I told her she was not, and it was very clear. I hope she claws upward and makes it back to the Games. Our team and the fans really enjoy her personality.

When I land in San Diego tonight, I'll go straight home and get some sleep. I have Julian Alcaraz coming over to Yarrow to test tomorrow. I'm going to have him test the stretched-out Amanda. I've decided to have him try the 13-11-9-7-5 version, and I might have him test a GHD/push press/ SkiErg test. I'm not really sold on the GHD test at this point, but I want to start experimenting with it to see what direction I should go. It will be a great official first day of testing.

When sitting at the Regional in Portland today, I thought it might be time to combine the West with California in one large West Regional. Maybe move Canada back to its own Regional, where it's just Canadian athletes versus Canadian athletes. The whole country at one Regional.

At the West Regional I also had a meeting with Amy Hicks about taking a look at the current regions and proposing a new plan with some guidance I gave her. I want an Asia Regional, a South America Regional, an Australia Regional and maybe two European events, and then we can take a look at the States, maybe combine a few. Apparently she has a background in statistics and is good with stuff like this, so I'm very interested in seeing what she proposes. I would never have sought her out for this had Justin not said she would be a great person to offer insight. I like to try new people with tasks like this. Hopefully she provides some useful analysis.

Change is good. Change is necessary to make our sport grow and to figure out where we belong. Not reckless change, but change that makes sense in ultimately supporting the test and the global nature of our sport. Yes, it's time South America and Asia have a Regional. Brazil has the second-largest number of CrossFit affiliates. Within the last year, it passed Canada, Australia and the U.K. to be second only to the U.S. That enthusiasm and growth almost demands a Regional for South America. Same thing with Asia, particularly China and Korea. We already have a very large presence in Korea and are growing fast in China, so it makes sense to at least look at having a Regional there. Maybe those areas don't get five spots but something like one to three spots. So different regions have different numbers of Games spots available. It's an interesting concept I would like to explore, and by explore

I mean having other people dive into it to make proposals, presentations and recommendations about what might make sense.

Finally, I'll end tonight's notes with the Reebok Nano 8.0 shoe, which I saw. I think the 8 looks great. It's not a huge departure from the 7 but has some improvements and a different weave. I think that's OK and probably better than reinventing the wheel every year or so as they have in the past.

I also learned from Kenny Gamble, our main point of contact at Reebok, that the Grace shoe—the women-only CrossFit shoe—has done great. Women love it. So Reebok is going to focus more on that and the Nano line. They're going to do away with the Speed variation, which doesn't bother me. I think that shoe was almost too specific to running, but that's just my personal opinion. I hope the new weave catches on. I think it's a great shoe and looks amazing, too.

I would really love to see Reebok do well. Who doesn't want to root for the underdog? Reebok's rival in this space—footwear for CrossFit—is the global behemoth Nike. If I were not a member of CrossFit HQ and just a regular CrossFit athlete, I would go with the Reebok shoe just because Nike is the big dog and Reebok is the underdog. Or maybe in that alternate life I would go with NOBULL. I don't like the name, but I like their female athletes, the Brookes, and I think their shoe looks cool.

*Saturday, June 3, 12:16 p.m.*
I met up with Julian Alcaraz today to test. It was a quick session without a lot of hang-out time or messing around. I told him what he was going to do—descending reps of ring muscle-ups and snatches—and he went straight to warming up for the test.

While he warmed up, his wife Miranda and I spoke about her pregnancy, and we watched the men do Event 3 at the Atlantic Regional. It was a great heat in which Noah slipped up toward the end and Ben Smith's time from the earlier heats remained the fastest. Miranda mentioned she hopes Ben's brother makes it. After Event 3, Alec is currently in second, so he's in great position to qualify for the Games for the first time.

A few minutes after that heat was done, Julian let me know he was ready to start. I gave him the countdown and he attacked the workout.

13-11-9-7-5 REPS OF:

MUSCLE-UPS

SQUAT SNATCHES (135 LB.)

Right out of the gate, he broke the first set of muscle-ups at 5. That actually surprised me. Then he did another set of 5 and finally finished the last of the 13 at 54 seconds. On his set of 13 snatches, he did the same breakdown (*sets of 5, 5 and 3*) and finished the round of 13 snatches at 2:01.

He then attacked his round of 11 with 3 sets and finished the work in those rounds at 4:36. Around this time, Miranda asked me what I thought guys would get on this event or what time I was shooting for. I said probably around 10 minutes. Julian was essentially entering the Amanda portion of the event, the 9-7-5 part, but he had already done an additional 24 reps of each movement. He finished the round of 9 at 7:13, the round of 7 at 10:32 and finally the round of 5 at 12:09.

His overall time was a little slower than I expected. Immediately following the effort, he was very gassed and went to his back—a good sign. A 135-lb. squat snatch is light for the guys these days. Most people don't even bother doing Amanda with 135 anymore. They increase the weight. But in a version like this, 135 is very appropriate. I asked Julian what he thought about it, and he said he thinks the best will for sure be under 10 minutes. I asked if he thought guys would go for unbroken first sets, and he said for sure.

After he rested 10 or 15 minutes, I had him experiment with some single-arm dumbbell push presses. He did some with 85 lb. and was able to cycle them at a steady pace. Then I had him try some with 100. He was able to move those, too, but it was obviously challenging. We discussed how he thinks that would feel for most, and he said it would work the little guys. I agree. Julian has a large frame and is really strong, but some of the little guys who have qualified for the Games might struggle with the 100-lb. dumbbell.

I think I might contact Matt Lodin and have him test the muscle-up workout tomorrow, just to get another angle on it. I like having multiple people test the same events, especially for the Games. Usually I don't tell the testers the other athletes' times or that anyone else tested it at all.

I just watched Ben Smith crush Event 4. There are two heats remaining, so a lot can still happen.

*5:34 p.m.*

I spent a few hours at Yarrow this evening. My mind was all over the place in between watching Regionals events and trying to program, but I had some productive moments. I started to sketch out another view I use to analyze what I program and consider what types of movements we're doing. Weightlifting movements are one category *(I include a subcategory of odd objects)*. Monostructural movements are another category—running, swimming, biking and the stuff that makes you breathe hard in the traditional sense. And finally gymnastics movements. I take a look at all the weekend's programming from a variety of perspectives, and the distribution of movement types is important.

For example, if I find I've programmed 20 weightlifting movements, 7 gymnastics movements and 4 monostructural movements, I have a very unbalanced test that is skewed toward loaded movements that favor the strongest guys. This wouldn't be a good way to find the Fittest on Earth.

I'll take a look at the number of movements in events. Is the competition just full of couplets and singles? Do I have variety in the structure of movements? I'll also look at rep schemes and take a global view of the time domains of the events. How many are short? How many are sprints? How many are medium and long? And so on.

Writing this out today helped me notice some things I might want to change already, which is good. That's the point. For example, on Saturday I have the SkiErg and the Assault bike in two different events. I have an aversion to that, but after taking the whole schedule into consideration, I might be comfortable with it.

While writing this stuff down on my whiteboards, I saw some notes I had to erase to make room for the new info. One was an interval event and the other was chaos. I still want to do chaos, but I don't know how or where yet. Possibly Saturday night. Another possibility for Saturday night: the interval idea. I've never really liked intervals as tests for the Games or Regionals, but I've never done intervals at this level, so maybe it's time to include one event in the programming. It would have to be super simple and easy to understand. At a quick glance, I think row for calories and max thrusters in 2 minutes, rest 1 minute, repeat 4 times. Row 20 calories and then use the remaining time for thrusters. I like this concept. I just have to test it out and see if those movements are right and if I like the way it plays out.

I also made some progress on Team Event 2 on Thursday—Amanda. I don't think I'm going to have them all do Amanda. Maybe I'll have them do 5 rounds of 4 muscle-ups and 4 squat snatches for one pair, then 5 and 5, and finally 6 and 6. The issue is that I want this event to highlight individual strengths or weaknesses, and I have it as a 30-minute heat, meaning a 25-minute time cap on work. If I go one athlete at a time, I have 4 minutes or so per person. I'll test the 5 rounds of 6 and 6 with Matt and see what his time is. If it's in the 4-minute window or so, it should be good. Well, that's essentially 4 minutes for Isabel and 30 muscle-ups. Maybe that's too aggressive. Maybe I should make a 3-rep version, a 4-rep version and a 5-rep version for 5 rounds each. I want 5 rounds because that's what I'm doing with the individuals. After seeing Julian's 5-round Amanda this morning, I'm pretty set on doing 5. I sent Bill a note this afternoon to prepare the five rigs—and we'll also need 50 short barbells for the snatches in this event.

This evening, Tim Chan sent me a blog post Talayna Fortunato wrote on the injuries at Regionals. I didn't read it, largely because a few weeks ago she had the audacity to text me and ask if I programmed this event to hurt people and expose those who might be juicing. That's such a ridiculous thing to accuse me of doing. I like Talayna, and she knows me better than that. No need for me to read what she posted about the programming.

A lot is said about me and the programming. If I read it all and listened to it all, it would probably drive me crazy. So to maintain my sanity, I tune out a lot and don't read or look at a lot of stuff. I need to keep the negativity away from me—especially at this stage.

*Sunday, June 4, 5:03 p.m.*
Didn't make it to Yarrow. Busy day at home and watching the final day of Regionals.

There was some great action today, with a lot of movement throughout the events. Ben made it back, so no problem there. Dave Eubanks was wrong, and I was wrong for doubting Ben. Poor Tia Wright from the West missed the Games again, and it all came down to the last event. And a former Army guy put on a great show and made it on the men's side. George Sanchez was in seventh and basically needed a victory on the final event. He made that happen, and it was a very exciting race.

Overall, I'm very happy with the Regionals and how the programming played out. I would have done some things differently. I would have made Individual Event 1 a little longer. Event 2 was fine. The injuries sucked, but the event didn't need to change. Event 3 was good. I liked how it played out. Event 4 I might have laid out differently. After Week 1 I hated it, after Week 2 I could tolerate it, and by Week 3 I appreciated it. But I could have laid it out better. Event 5 I liked. I could have used a squat snatch instead, but I was happy with how this one played out. I'm happy with Event 6 and how it played out, but if I were to program this one again, I would use standard box jumps. I think that would have made it better. But I'm not unhappy with how we did this one. It was a good learning opportunity for us and the community.

Although I didn't make it into Yarrow today, I had some good thoughts about some of the programming. I did the CrossFit.com workout of the day today, and it was Fight Gone Bad-style: 5 rounds of 1 minute of sumo deadlift high pulls, 1 minute of push presses, 1 minute of rowing and 1 minute of rest. It made me think about the interval event I might do at the Games. I think three components might be good. Rowing, bar muscle-ups and then something loaded, like cleans. I don't know if this one will make the cut, but I'm going to experiment with it and see if it can get to a place where I'm happy with it.

This evening, I'm going to watch Game 2 of the NBA Finals. I grew up in the Bay Area and was actually a Warriors fan when they were really bad, but that didn't continue as I grew up, even when they started winning. I initially hated LeBron James, especially after The Decision, but I've grown to really appreciate how good and how dominant he is. So I'm actually pulling for the Cavs. But really I'm hoping for a good series more than anything else because the rest of the playoffs really sucked.

*Monday, June 5, 9:56 a.m.*
I'm thinking about doing the event with the GHD, SkiErg and push presses in 2 sets now instead of 3. It has to be done east to west on the floor with two heats of 20, so that's one reason to avoid barbells. I'm currently thinking maybe 50 GHD reps, 40-30 SkiErg calories and then 30-10 push presses. Two rounds of that.

Matt Lodin is here at Yarrow warming up right now. I'm going to have him test what might be Team Event 2. It was supposed to be Amanda, but

I'm going to have five rigs in Madison, so I want to use all of them. I could stretch it out for the teams, too, but only one person is going to be working at a time, I have 25 minutes to play with, and 25 divided by 6 equals about 4 minutes. So I need it to be fast. I'm thinking one pair does 5 squat snatches and 5 muscle-ups for 5 rounds, another pair does 4/4 for 5 rounds, and a final pairing does 3/3 for 5 rounds. When I say pair, I mean one male and one female, and they won't be working together. It will be individual efforts.

Another option I just thought of: 7-6-5-4-3 for 1 set, 6-5-4-3-2 for another and finally 5-4-3-2-1 for the last set. I'll see how the testing of the 5-5 for 5 goes with Matt.

*10:36 a.m.*

5 ROUNDS OF:

5 MUSCLE-UPS

5 SQUAT SNATCHES (135 LB.)

Matt took 5:45 to complete the 5-round variation. Of note, his first round was 40 seconds. In Round 2, he started breaking his snatches into 2 sets, and by Round 3 he was breaking up his muscle-ups into 2 sets. He did his final round of snatches unbroken. It looked taxing, and he was breathing very hard by the end. I actually liked how it played out. He said the top guys would for sure be under 5 minutes. So the 3-3 version should take around 3 minutes, the 4-4 version should take 4, and this one should take 5. That gives me 12 minutes for one gender and puts teams in the 24-minute realm if these assumptions are correct. The best teams should be in the range of 22 or 23 minutes, and about half the teams will hit the time cap. I like this direction. It might be a good test. It's a sprint with two movements teams didn't see at Regionals, and it will definitely highlight individual weaknesses—either in the squat snatch or the ring muscle-ups.

*3:36 p.m.*

I came in after lunch and got distracted by some sewing projects. Kinda wasted my time sewing instead of programming. I tried walking back in to program, but my mind was already elsewhere. I left Yarrow, went to Starbucks for a cold brew, went home, said hi to my family, had a snack and just returned for a programming session.

Earlier today, I had an idea while I was doing some other work. What about a Worm event in which the team holds the Worm while one to three members go off and do some other work? There is some good that might come out of that idea. I just need to play with it some more.

As I was driving over, I had another idea that might stick: 17.5 as a Games event scaled for Games competitors—something with 135-lb. thrusters and double-unders. Maybe with the Zeus rope. Ten rounds would be insane. Maybe less rounds, maybe the same. I like continuing themes, and this is a great way to do it. Maybe this idea will make it. I'm going to put it on my board of ideas.

*4:30 p.m.*

I also played around with the schedule a little, Sunday's in particular. I then laid out more of the analysis boards. Today I put up a list of types of events—singles, couplets, triplets, etc.—and another board that shows the ways they are combined.

I sat around a lot thinking about different events and workouts. I want to do the clean ladder on Saturday, and I thought about ways to make it unique. Maybe I could add burpees. Then I thought about HSPU with the clean ladder. Interestingly, we could use HSPU as a tiebreaker. Maybe once people fail at a weight, they go back to the wall and do HSPU to break ties with others who failed at the same weight.

I still have a lot of events to plan, and I felt like I made good progress. I know I'm ahead of schedule compared to years past, but with the Games in a new location with a new format, I still feel really behind. Well, I feel behind at this moment.

*5:51 p.m.*

Today I found out that Christian Lucero's testosterone levels tested very high, so they are taking things to the next round of testing. If he pops, we notify him and give him the option to appeal. If he appeals, we look at the appeal and take it from there. But we can't announce anything until that process is done or unless he decides to announce something on his own. Maybe he will blame it on some special mix of Progenex that he was taking or testing for that company. Wouldn't that be funny.

*Tuesday, June 6, 2:45 p.m.*

This morning I had Julian over to test again. I'm beginning to enjoy his company, and it's cool to get to know him better. Before testing, we hung out and shot the shit. He mentioned bringing his grill next time and cooking some tacos while we work out. Then he suggested some knockout before testing. I love knockout, so that was a no-brainer. I sucked. He and Stephane did great.

Then I had him warm up for the GHD/SkiErg/push-press test. I have this penciled in for Friday afternoon, after the O-course but before the 1RM snatch. I have it set for 20 athletes at a time, so we have limited space. I wanted to avoid more hip opening and pulling from the ground, so I'm testing a single-arm dumbbell push press.

2 ROUNDS OF:

50 GHD SIT-UPS

50 SKIERG CALORIES

10 PUSH PRESSES WITH A 100-LB. DUMBBELL

Julian started the test and finished the 50 GHD sit-ups in just under 2 minutes. Then he hit 50 calories on the SkiErg in about 2:40. He ripped the 100-lb. dumbbell off the floor and did 10 push presses in about 20 seconds for a Round 1 time of 4:44. As he got on the GHD and started the second round, I had seen enough to know I would make some changes. I quite often change the test in the middle because I saw something I didn't like or something I could improve.

I let him finish the second set of 50 GHDs, and it took about 2 minutes. As he started the SkiErg, I told him to do 40 calories instead. That took him about 2:20. When he got back to the dumbbell, I told him to do 20 reps total, switching arms every 5. That portion took him about 1 minute. He broke after every 5, putting the dumbbell on the ground after each set. I liked the second round much better.

Looking at it, I'm thinking I might program 50 GHDs, 30 calories and 20 push presses for 2 rounds. The SkiErg combines nicely with the GHD. You have two aggressive closings of the hips, but in different fashions. One closing is done with anchored feet, and the other is done from a standing position while pulling down on the cords of the SkiErg. Then we have a nice, heavy single-arm push press to finish off.

Julian mentioned that the GHD-SkiErg combo hurt because the GHD uses so much leg that it's tough to go straight into a pull that also uses a lot of leg. I liked the visual, too: He was laid out on the floor like roadkill. This one seemed to have a good bite.

I plan on running the 1RM snatch two or three hours later, and that's a concern. I asked him if he thought the push presses taxed his arms and would affect his ability to snatch. He said he didn't think so. I also asked him what he thought about how it would affect the little guys. He thinks it will be tough but they will be able to do it. I agree. It will be tough for guys like Josh Bridges and Cody Anderson, but the reps are not too crazy. And this is the Games. They should be able to handle it.

After we finished that, we let him rest before I had him play with the Banger. We laid it on the ground and had him hit it 25 feet. It took almost 2 minutes. Then we created an elevated platform to stand on, much like they do for firefighters in their challenge. Doing it that way took him a little more than 2 minutes, but it put him in a much better striking position. He mentioned that if he had to go 50 feet, that position would work much better. My original intent was to use the Assault bike and then the Banger for 50 feet. But at his pace—and if he didn't slow down—the Banger would take about 4-5 minutes for 50 feet, not including the bike.

I want this test to be about 3-4 minutes total, just a gut-check sprint. I texted Bill to ask if he can make a lighter version of the Banger. That way I can make it a sprint. I also realized I probably won't have the space for heats of 20. For safety, I need more room between athletes swinging hammers. So we might have to do heats of 14, 14 and 13.

I've also been thinking a lot about the Team Amanda workout. I was leaning toward 5 rounds of 5-5, 4-4 and 3-3, but today I had an idea that places more emphasis on the muscle-ups: Keep all rounds at 5 muscle-ups and only change the number of squat snatches. So 5 rounds of 5-3, 5-4 and 5-5. I might have Matt test 5 rounds of 5-3 tomorrow.

*4:13 p.m.*

My mind has been all over the place this afternoon. I tweaked the schedule to accommodate three heats per gender on the Banger. I also did some work organizing the events on my whiteboard. I keep thinking about the test that crossed my mind earlier today while driving: 17.5 at 135/95 lb.

Honestly, it almost sounds too brutal. It might be too hard. Too much volume, too many heavy thrusters. The thing is these competitors are good—very good. I could have Julian test it on Friday. If it gets ugly and just takes too long, I could cut it off. I'm really curious about how it will go down and look. And I like the idea of bringing that Open workout to the Games as a final event of a day or a final-day event. I need to process this some more. It's hard to get out of my mind.

I actually just had another idea I need to write down now. It's a variant of an event we did a few years ago: handstand push-ups and walking lunges with four different weights or loads. So do 1 round of HSPU, then lunge with one weight. Then do the next round of HSPU and lunge the next load. And so on. We did something like this with handstand push-ups and sled pulls. It could make for an exciting event. Going to write it on the board.

*4:21 p.m.*

I took that idea to the board and morphed it into something different: HSPU into handstand walks. HSPU into lunges. HSPU into pulls. HSPU into pushes? Hmm. I don't know where this is going, but I like it.

*Wednesday, June 7, 8:39 a.m.*

I came into Yarrow earlier than normal. I usually work out at this time. But it's a rest day, so I'm coming in to get ready for testing this afternoon and to make some progress before that session. I have an HQ meeting in Santa Cruz next week, and I'm dreading it. The last thing I want to do right now is leave San Diego. I really need to dig into this uninterrupted. Hopefully I can make some good progress over the course of the next few days. I think I can. I just need to play with it and continue pushing on.

*9:15 a.m.*

I put the heavy 17.5 on the schedule for Sunday, but as I looked at it, it might fit better as Saturday's final event. I moved it there. I also continued to think about the final three-part event. It's very similar to The Cinco 1 and 2 from 2013. What's interesting about The Cinco is that I planned those events literally the night before and the morning of the final day of the Games. That's how Games programming used to happen. Some stuff wasn't finished until the Games were already in progress. These days, I have strict TV deadlines and other considerations, but with Yarrow I'm pretty much able to figure everything out before the Games. Sometimes stuff that is not tested requires odd objects we use for the first time when they arrive at the Games.

I also gave some thought to the clean ladder. In 2016, we had a squat-clean ladder. We had them do 10 reps at 245 lb., 8 at 265, 6 at 285, 4 at 305 and 2 at 325, and 31 of the athletes finished it. Nine didn't. So I was thinking about doing something similar but different: take the weights up, make it heavier and add a second movement. I was thinking pull-ups. I sketched out this event: 20 pull-ups, 2 cleans at 225, 20 pull-ups, 2 cleans at 245, 20 pull-ups, 2 cleans at 265, 20 pull-ups, 2 cleans at 285, 20 pull-ups, 2 cleans at 305, 20 pull-ups, 2 cleans at 325, 20 pull-ups, 2 cleans at 345, 20 pull-ups, 2 cleans at 365. I like that, but it's a ton of pull-ups. Maybe I'll drop the pull-ups down to 15 or 16. I like the way this will play out. Maybe I'll have Julian test it this weekend or early next week.

I'm going to step away this morning to get some shooting in at the indoor range. I haven't done that in a while, and I need a break from this. With all the ammo Federal Premium Ammunition has provided for me, I have no excuse not to go shoot.

*4:19 p.m.*
Earlier today, I had a couple of testing sessions go down separately. At 1:15, I had Tommy Pease come over and go through the same GHD/SkiErg/push-press test I had Julian do a few days ago.

I changed Julian's reps in the middle of the workout, but I had the reps set for Tommy. I told him to do 50 GHDs, 40 SkiErg calories and 20 push presses with a 100-lb. dumbbell, changing arms every 5 reps.

Tommy is a small guy. He's on the shorter end and weighs about 170. He was once a great athlete in the SoCal scene. He missed qualifying for the Games two years in a row. He's not as good as he used to be, but he's still in amazing shape. He's tested Games workouts for me in the past. One of the memorable events he tested was Naughty Nancy, a variation of Nancy with increased OHS weight, reps and running distance.

While Tommy was warming up, it was very obvious the 100-lb. dumbbell was going to be challenging for him. He struggled with it on his right arm and at first could not get any on his left arm. After a tad more practice, he was able to knock some out on the left arm. So we decided to proceed as written.

**2 ROUNDS OF:**

**50 GHD SIT-UPS**

**50 SKIERG CALORIES**

**20 PUSH PRESSES WITH A 100-LB. DUMBBELL**

It started off great. His GHD set was a little bit faster than Julian's, and his set on the SkiErg was a bit slower—but not much. He got to the push presses around 5 minutes. Julian had to do a set of 20 push presses to complete his second round, and he finished 20 reps in 4 sets in a little over a minute. Tommy's first round didn't go so well. On his first right-arm set, he did 4 and then put it down. He had to pick it back up to finish the fifth rep. He did his first 5 left-arm reps in 3 very difficult sets. His second 5 right-arm reps also took 2 sets, and then his final left-arm reps took 3 rough sets. All of this took about 5 minutes, and he was worked. I actually considered stopping the workout there. I really didn't need to see more, but I decided to let him finish strong. His second round of GHDs started very slowly, and then at about 10 he said he needed to stop. I said, "Yeah, go ahead. *Don't worry about it.*" So he stopped the test. He mentioned feeling lightheaded, and he said he really doesn't train high-rep GHDs right now.

We discussed how the 100-lb. dumbbell felt, and he said it was hard but seems appropriate for the smaller guys at the Games. Obviously, things at the Games are hard. If you make it to the Games as a smaller athlete, you often have a disadvantage with loaded things. On the other side of the discussion, you often have an easier time with unloaded movements.

I think the test was a success. I wanted to see a smaller guy handle the 100-lb. dumbbell. I saw that, and it was very hard for Tommy. But he didn't qualify for the Games, so I feel confident the loading is appropriate in the rep scheme I want to use.

After Tommy left, Matt showed up. I had Matt test the Team Amanda variation that has the muscle-ups fixed at 5 for 5 rounds, with just the snatches changing. I had him test 5 rounds of 5 muscle-ups and 3 squat snatches at 135 lb. He started off very fast and finished 2 rounds in about a minute. Then it got a little slower. On rounds 4 and 5, he had to break up the muscle-ups, and he ended up finishing at 4:12. That has me thinking 25 reps for everyone might be too much. This version would be the "*low*" variation, so the medium variation would take around 5 minutes. The high variation Matt tested was over 5. With six people going through, I have to remember I have an average of about 4 minutes for each person. We decided to have Matt come back tomorrow to test 5 rounds of 3 and 3 just to see how fast it is and how he feels. He thinks it will be too easy. It might be, but I'm OK with that. Some of these sprints are not necessarily super hard but require you to push. We'll find out more tomorrow.

Today I actually feel I'm in a pretty good place with the programming. It feels like things are coming together—well, for the individuals. I haven't done much for the teams. But the key is to make the Individual competition great and something I'm proud to present to the world. Then I can focus on making the Team events great. But understand that I do have some Team events done already. It's just that the focus now is Individual programming.

*Thursday, June 8, 3:28 p.m.*
Last night Justin hit me up and said we have to run the individuals during a specific hour on Saturday because of our live-TV window. That could mean a lot of changes, and I spent some time adjusting the schedule to accommodate that.

I met Matt at Yarrow at 10 a.m. to have him test another variant of the Team muscle-up/snatch event. This is the third time in about 5 days that he's done a variant of this event. Today he tested one of my original ideas, which might be the shortest of the events.

### 5 ROUNDS OF:

### 3 MUSCLE-UPS

### 3 SNATCHES (135 LB.)

Obviously, it was very fast. He did it in 2:42, and it had him breathing hard. He took a couple of short breaks before the fourth and fifth sets of muscle-ups. It could be even shorter if he didn't rest. Matt thinks it might be too few reps, but I actually like it. It's still a tough challenge. The team event could look like this:

*One male and one female do 5 rounds of 3 muscle-ups and 3 snatches*

*One male and one female do 5 rounds of 4 muscle-ups and 4 snatches*

*One male and one female do 5 rounds of 5 muscle-ups and 5 snatches*

They all get a sprint in, and there's an opportunity for some strategy in figuring out who does what version. Even with these variations, it will be a lot of work for teams to finish under the time cap of 25 minutes. It could be worth trying. At this moment, I'm planning on this version, and I'm actually excited about it.

*5:19 p.m.*

I worked some more on the potential clean ladder with pull-ups. I might have Julian test that early next week or this weekend if he can. I dropped the reps to 16 instead of 20. Sixteen reps per round will produce 128 reps over 8 rounds—less volume.

A couple of issues come to mind with that high rep count. Right now, I have the test in an 8-minute window. That's probably way too tight—but maybe not. It takes less than 30 seconds for 16 pull-ups, and 2 cleans at the early weights will be fast. Maybe it will take 40-45 seconds for the first few rounds, and then they slow down a little as they get to the rounds with the heavier loads. I'll test to figure this stuff out.

Julian will be a perfect guy for testing because he's among the stronger Games athletes.

Another issue I have is the volume. In the Open, they did way more pull-ups in 17.3, but that was the only thing we dictated to them that week. The rest of their training and workouts were their own. Here at the Games, we are dictating their schedule and their volume. I think 160 might be too many pull-ups considering what else they have going on. But I'll see how they affect Julian and what his time is.

I also worked on Saturday's schedule for CBS a little more. TV requirements are essentially causing me to change Saturday a lot, and I'm going to have to rethink how I do the Team clean. I originally had the Team women going, then the Individual women, with both groups using the same setup. We would do a big transition, then Team men and Individual men would go. But because of CBS' requirements, I have to change. So now it will be a group effort with all six athletes. I don't know what it's going to look like yet, but I'll figure it out soon.

Thursday's schedule is mostly done. Friday is almost there. Saturday is coming together. For Sunday, I have some ideas, but there are also some points at which things are not falling in place. I like the idea of a rope-climb event in the stadium, but I'm having trouble figuring out how I can plug that into Sunday and still maintain a wide-open floor for the finale I want to experiment with—the event with a handstand walk, lunges and maybe a pull.

Tomorrow is a big test day. Matt and Julian are coming. I'll have Matt test the GHD/SkiErg/push-press workout, and I'll have Julian test 17.5 at 135 lb. I'm very interested in seeing how that treats him.

I experimented with one last thing today at Yarrow, and I found I really like laying out the bars horizontally in line with the lanes. This setup would be used to lay out multiple bars of ascending weight. Once an athlete gets to the bar, he or she spins it to the typical setup perpendicular to the lane. For workouts with a lot of bars, where the weights are ascending, or where the athlete leaves the bar to do other work and returns later, it allows the fans to glance at the floor and see who is further along or who is struggling. The bars will let you know where the athlete is in the workout.

*Friday, June 9, 2:29 p.m.*
Today was a good day of testing. We met Julian at Yarrow at 10 a.m. The first thing he did was pull out his Traeger grill and some food. He started prepping meat and potatoes to throw on the grill while he tested. After his prep was done, I briefed him on the test. It was also the first time Stephane had heard it.

When I said *"17.5 but with 135,"* the looks on their faces were priceless. I imagine the Games athletes will have similar looks when I announce this to them, too. Julian was very excited to tackle this one. He had a great attitude during his warm-up and was very excited to do this version of 17.5.

10 ROUNDS OF:

9 THRUSTERS (135 LB.)

35 DOUBLE-UNDERS

He started with a great pace, and his first full round was complete in 43 seconds.

He broke up his third set of double-unders into 2 sets, and he completed 3 rounds in 2:36. At that point, I was thinking he might go sub 10.

He finished 5 rounds in 4:49, and I knew sub 10 would be hard because his pace would slow.

He finished Round 10 at 11:29. I was very impressed.

Julian broke the double-unders up in 7 of the 10 rounds, and he broke the final round of thrusters into 2 sets: 7 thrusters, drop the bar, then 2 more. Every other thruster round had looked steady and solid. He did 90 thrusters at 135 and 350 double-unders in 11:29.

He was, of course, laid out and writhing in pain. Once he recovered, I asked him what he thought the top guys will do. He said low 10s, with possibly an athlete or two under 10. I agreed. Seeing this one go down—and seeing how well he handled 135—made me believe this is more than appropriate for the Games athletes and will be a great event on Saturday night. I can already see it going down. I can see how I'll announce it to them on the floor, and then they'll attack it 30 minutes or so later. This one has me very excited.

After the testing, I called Roger from Assault over. He came down and we had some epic games of knockout. Then we had some awesome smoked strip steak and potatoes. Julian is a good cook—he also owns Fierro's Kitchen, a business that makes meals for Orange County affiliates. More importantly, as I spend more time with Julian and get to know him, I'm learning he's also a really good guy. It's hard for people to come into my circle or for me to like people right away. I'm very standoffish with people, and I keep them at arm's length when I first meet them. But I like Julian, and I enjoy his company.

I need to go buy some hay bales. I'll probably do that this weekend.

*Saturday, June 10, 6:42 p.m.*
I didn't do much today at Yarrow with regard to programming, but I did get a couple of interesting new things. I went to a cattle feed store in Encinitas and purchased three bales of hay—straw, actually. While I was there, I watched the worker load them up with the hay hooks. He made it look so effortless, and it looked like a great piece of equipment to use in an event. Maybe move 20 bales from one side of the field to the other. I think it

would be cool, but as I imagine it, I come to scenarios in which athletes are running with those things, slipping and falling and putting hooks through their faces or into their bodies. That would not be good. But the thought of using them has stayed in my mind for now.

I took the three bales of hay to Yarrow and stacked them up. I did a couple of burpee box jump-overs. The barrier was high. Then I tried a couple of box jumps. The stack was really high for that. I was able to do the box jumps, which actually surprised me. But it was interesting because they are only stacked up, not secured together. I like the hay-bale idea for an event. I have to program something with the bales, most likely a 400-m run and some burpees over the bales. Maybe they clean an item over and then burpee over the bales. I don't know yet, but I'll play with it. I still had the hay-hook idea in the back of my head when I left Yarrow and headed home.

A few hours later, my brother Kenny showed up. Kenny is older by seven years, and he works for Rogue. He's at the Games and Regionals every year. He had driven down from The Ranch with his family to go to Disneyland. He brought the original slide for the Banger, so now I can test to see how it works on that. When we played around with the event the first time, we just set the Banger on the concrete floor.

I showed him the bales of hay and mentioned how I might use them.

*"What if we used hay hooks?"* I said.

*"No way. It's too dangerous,"* he said.

He then went on to tell me a story of how he was doing a workout with hay hooks and hay bales. At one point, the hook pulled through the hay and stabbed him in the chest. Yikes. I'm definitely going to scratch that plan. Again, the last thing I need is athletes' impaling themselves with hay hooks at the CrossFit Games.

*Sunday, June 11, 8:15 a.m.*
My mind has been bouncing all over the place this morning, really for the past 12 hours. I had some ideas this morning, so I came into Yarrow to flesh them out. The hay-bale combo of a clean and burpee over the top is really solidifying in my mind. I think it's a good combo that could have a bite to it. I was thinking of combining that with an even shorter run. Not 400, but maybe 200 or 300. Something like 4-6 rounds of run 200-400 meters

and 10 cleans over the obstacle and burpees over the obstacle. I'm going to work on that this morning.

The other idea I had floating around was changing the clean/pull-up workout. As of right now, we have a ton of couplets. I need to add some balance, so maybe I can make that a triplet by altering the pull-up section to include pull-ups and toes-to-bars. Something like 10 pull-ups, 8 toes-to-bars and 2 cleans *(weight ascending)* for 8 rounds. I'm going to start sketching some of these ideas out on my paper pad.

*8:50 a.m.*

The north-lot floor is the outdoor venue we are creating next to the obstacle course, and it's essentially a smaller version of the soccer field from Carson. This is where we'll do the run/hay-bale event if it makes the cut. I played with some options and came to a point where I have something I would like to have tested by Matt or Julian. I could have Matt test this one because it's not so technical or difficult. It's just really a *"go"* event that asks how hard you want to push. Here's the version I came up with:

**5 ROUNDS OF:**

**RUN 400 METERS**

**10 CLEANS OVER THE HAY BALES PLUS BURPEES OVER THE BALES**

This would be laid out across the north-lot floor. So on the start signal, they would run 400 meters to get back to their first set of hay bales. They would do 10 cleans plus burpees over the hay. And then on the 10th rep they would advance the object to the next set of bales. They would repeat this 5 times. After the fifth set, they would either carry the object across the finish line or just sprint across.

I want to do heats of 20 on this, and each person needs six bales of hay to build each wall section. Women will probably get four bales. So 6 x 20 athletes is 120, and 120 x 5 rounds is 600. I texted J-Mac and said we will need 600 bales of hay. At roughly $10 a bale, that's $6,000 in hay. Not a big deal. It will make for a great event.

I'm also considering just making it a burpee over the hay, but then I would increase the burpee reps. Right now, I have this as an 18-minute heat. Maybe I'll make it 20. A 400-meter run in something like this is roughly 1:45, and I think 10 clean burpees will take under a minute. So call it 3 minutes per round and 15 minutes for 5 rounds. So this test should take anywhere between 14 and 17 minutes. I should be able to have someone test this soon so I can figure it out.

On the clean workout, I'm making it 8 rounds of 8 chest-to-bar pull-ups, 8 toes-to-bars and 2 cleans, with the weight increasing each round. I'll test that tomorrow with Julian. He said his 1RM clean is 375, so it's very unlikely he'll finish it, but that's OK. I'll see how far he gets and how long it takes.

*1:21 p.m.*

I'm considering moving Saturday's run/hay-bale workout to Sunday because I currently have it as Saturday morning's test, and it has an odd-object clean. The next event has barbell cleans. Generally, I hate that type of redundancy. Even though they're different cleans, they're still cleans. I'll see what I can do about that. I can change things by moving the test to the Sunday spot or removing the clean. But taking the object over the hay is such a nice touch and something we haven't done before, so maybe I can live with the back-to-back cleans. I do think the barbell clean and med-ball clean are very different. But I'm just trying to convince myself that the redundancy is OK.

I just had another idea: Move the snatch from Friday to Saturday, and move this event to Friday from Saturday.

Another idea is to just make the barbell clean a heavy deadlift. I just penciled out some possibilities for that option: 405, 425, 445, 465, 485, 505, 525, 545. At last year's Games, eight athletes lifted 545 or more, 16 lifted 525 or more, and 27 did 505 or more. Josh Bridges did 475, which would be past the fourth bar in this setup.

But the clean would make for a much more exciting event. I'm leaning toward that movement. I still plan on having someone test the barbell-clean version tomorrow to see what I think of it.

*5:23 p.m.*

I came in this evening because I feel like I'm running out of time. I started off by playing basketball. It usually helps me to come in and ground with something instead of going straight into programming. This is not a rule, but often I need to shoot, hit the speed bag or sew for a few minutes before diving into the work. Once I was satisfied with my shooting practice, I dove into the programming with no real goal.

I first started by updating my boards that allow me to analyze all the programming. I then made a list of what movements have not been used or are not plugged in yet. This reminded me that I need to do this for the time domains, too. I think I might be heavy on medium-length events and don't have enough sprints. I will play that out and see.

All this made me think of Sunday's north-lot work event. I started jotting down some ideas and movements. I listed a bear-hug carry, a grip carry, a drag and finally a yoke. I started playing out how it could look. Take each object one length down, run back and grab another in order. Once you take the last one across the line, time stops. But then I started imagining the reset time—it would be horrible. Bingo! I will make them take the objects down and back!

Here's how that could look: You have all four objects on one side, and you have to get them to the other side. Once they are all there, you take them back to the beginning. A cool twist here is that we will not dictate the order. Athletes can pick the order of implements. That will play nicely. Because we are going down and back, I'll reduce the loads. Conceptually, I like this. It will be fun and interesting to see which strategies they use.

Then I started thinking about the finale and what we could do there. I thought of a handstand-push-up/rowing event. This would be very cool: 21-15-9 HSPU and rowing for calories. Great combo, nice format, nasty sprint. I like that test. Maybe I'll try to plug it in one of our other events.

Coming back to the finale, I was plugging in HSPU with a rope pull, HSPU with lunges, HSPU with handstand walks. Just notes and ideas on the board at this time.

What's interesting is that last year I had the final done early. It was an anchor everything else was kind of built around. The concept of the thruster and pegboard was one of the first ideas I had planned for the Games last year, besides the repeat of Murph. The actual final product took a while to get to, and I went through a lot of testing to create a variation that was doable in a decent time. But this year I have almost every day programmed but the final, which is not completely unusual. There have been years when I programmed Sunday on Sunday morning, so I guess this is better than that.

But I'm sensitive this year to the final. I want it to be great. We have had great finals and some that were not so great. Last year's final was a great event and test. I love the programming, but it wasn't the most exciting final. This year I'm going to try to make the final exciting. I know the formula, the recipe. We use it every year in Regionals. I just need to follow that. Maybe that's what I need to keep telling myself: *"Fuck all this complex stuff I'm thinking about now. Just make it raw and keep it real CrossFit. Keep it true to who we are and who I am."*

*Monday, June 12, 12:35 p.m.*

We had a good day of testing. I had Matt and Julian come in. Julian was running a little late, so I had Matt start off and test the GHD/SkiErg/push-press event. I had him do this:

2 ROUNDS OF:

50 GHDS

30 SKIERG CALORIES (I DROPPED IT TO 30 FROM 40)

20 PUSH PRESSES WITH A 100-LB. DUMBBELL

He got through the first round pretty fast and only put the dumbbell down once, after doing 15 unbroken–including a mandatory arm switch after every 5 reps. I actually don't think that's a good strategy for someone his size, but we'll see at the Games. On his second round, he actually stopped twice on the GHD, which surprised me. But it is a lot of reps. He then pushed through the SkiErg and got back to the final set of push presses/jerks. He ended up doing those in 3 sets, starting with his left arm, which turned out to be a good strategy. He went left *(his weak arm)*, right, left, right. He put it down after 5 and 10 but switched to finish the last 10 reps. His time was 12:05.

I have it as a 15-minute heat, with a 12-minute cap as of right now. I could make that 13, and then there would be plenty of time. It's heats of 20, so maybe keeping it at 12 is better because it gives more time for everyone to set up. This was the third time I had this one tested. I might have it tested again, but not in the immediate future. Maybe in a few weeks.

Next, I had Julian warm up for the clean event:

8 ROUNDS OF:

8 CHEST-TO-BAR PULL-UPS

8 TOES-TO-BARS

2 CLEANS (225, 245, 265, 285, 305, 325, 345, 365 LB.)

He started out fast and finished the first round in 37 seconds.

The second round was finished at 1:36.

He finished the third round (*2 cleans at 265*) at 2:40.

In the fourth round (*2 cleans at 285*), he finished at 4:02. Of note, he broke up the toes-to-bars for the first time.

On the 5th round (*2 cleans at 305*), he again broke the toes-to-bars once, and he went for a power clean on the first rep at 305, but it morphed into a squat clean. The second rep was a true squat clean. The rest of his cleans all used the squat. He finished this round at 5:41.

On Round 6 (*2 cleans at 325*), he broke up the pull-ups and toes-to-bars. He hit the first clean at the 7:19 mark and locked out the second at 7:43. He looked very strong at this point.

The seventh round had a 345-lb. bar. I knew Julian's max clean was around 370, so this was getting up there. He again broke the pull-ups and the toes-to-bars into 2 sets, then stuck the 345 clean at 9:30. He nailed the second one 41 seconds later and finished the round at 10:11.

On the final round, he broke the pull-ups into 2 sets and the toes-to-bars into 3 sets. He finished that part of the workout at 11:31, then rested 40 seconds before making his first attempt at 365. He set up and then pulled fast, reversing direction to land underneath the weight. He made one good attempt to stand it up but quickly dropped the load. He was visibly disappointed and paced around a little, then decided he would make another attempt. He tried again at the 13-minute mark but just deadlifted and stopped.

I was very proud of his effort. He was the perfect guy to test this for me. He is a very strong CrossFit athlete—not the strongest, like Fraser and Froning and the Andersons and Smiths, but one level below those athletes and much stronger than those I would consider the weaker ones in the field.

I'm thinking about either reducing the reps on the pull-ups/toes-to-bars combo or just making the pull-ups regular pull-ups to speed things up and make it more about the strength test. Ultimately, this is a strength test with some annoying body-weight movements in the middle. I don't know if the final version will look like this, but I like where it's going.

After that we played some great games of knockout. I won some, and I lost a bunch. Julian probably won the most. But today everybody at least got one or two wins.

We then played with the Banger. We have a 10-foot section of the slide it sits in, so we did 10 feet for time. We had Julian go first, and he did it in about 1 minute. I asked Matt to go next, and he did it in 52 seconds. Then I decided to take a shot at it. I did it in 47 seconds! I was stoked about that. Next, I asked Marston Sawyers to do it—he's in town filming. It took over a minute. His technique was so bad. He really didn't know what he was doing. It was pretty funny.

After that we discussed technique a little, and Julian decided to do it again. He also wore gloves on the second attempt. It took him 37 seconds! He crushed my time, as he should, considering he's 20 lb. heavier than me and a Games-level athlete.

My original thoughts had been to have them do 50 feet, but after all this testing I'm thinking 20-25 feet would be more appropriate. Matt suggested something interesting: He said I could get a heavier dead-blow hammer. The one we are using is 10 lb., and a heavier hammer will make it faster. I'll have Stephane purchase some heavier tools so we can experiment.

*3:46 p.m.*
Our Stanley hammer was brutal on our hands. It has a bunch of texture to it. So I just researched some other brands and hammers. I found a couple of other brands that make 12-lb. hammers, 2 lb. over the weight of the current hammer, and it looks like the handles are smooth, which should be more forgiving on the hands. I sent the links to Stephane and told him to order a 9 and a 12 of each brand so we can decide what we want to use.

I also thought of some other variants of this test. It would be cool to do 2 rounds. Assault bike 30, 10 feet of hammer, 2 rounds for time. But in the way I want to do this, it would require a fuck-ton of gear—40 slides and 40 Bangers. I asked Bill what he thought about that, and he said he could do it, but he would prefer if we did a version that used less gear. So I could settle on an Assault bike for 30 calories, do 20 feet on the Banger and then another 30 calories on the bike. Or something like that.

Regardless, this event will favor larger athletes and those who have worked with hammers before. But I'm OK with those compromises.

*4:26 p.m.*
I'm having doubts about using 17.5++ as the Saturday-night event. Two things are causing these doubts. I wonder if I should do a faster event there, a sprint, because that's three longer events that day—well, the longer run event on the north lot, the clean and jerk at 8-12 minutes, and 17.5++ at 8-12 minutes, too. So I wonder if I should have a test of 2-4 minutes there.

The other thing is Julian said it made his legs very sore the next day. It's a lot of volume. Yes, I'm concerned about how much I take out of their legs for Sunday. I don't anticipate doing high volume on Sunday, so maybe it will be OK. It is the Games, after all. I think it will make an epic Saturday-night event, and it would make a great midday event on Sunday, but it just won't be the same as a Saturday-night finale.

*Tuesday, June 13, 5:06 p.m.*
I'm currently flying with our pilot, Mike Buttenob, and Rita Robinson, Maggie Glassman's mom, up to Scotts Valley. I have some planning meetings with the team at the HQ office this week. The timing is horrible. The last thing I want to do right now is break away from my cycle and routine of programming and testing at Yarrow. But I have to do this meeting with some of the other CrossFit execs—Jeff Cain, Bruce Edwards, Kathy Glassman, Nicole Carroll and Sevan Matossian. I think I will be able to see Greg, too.

My goal is to get what we need to get done tomorrow and hopefully be able to come home tomorrow night. If that doesn't happen, I won't be able to come home until Thursday evening, which would be less than ideal. On April 6, it was on this same flight in this same plane that I decided to start writing this log of my Games programming.

Last night I slept badly, which is uncommon. I am a good sleeper—I would say even a great sleeper. I'm usually out the moment I lie down and, when home, I'm up nine hours later. On the road, I almost never get that much sleep. At the Games, even less. But last night I couldn't fall asleep. I couldn't stop thinking about the Games and the events. I thought about the doubts I'm having with the events, and I considered changing some of the tests. I think it was an hour before I finally fell asleep. I ended up waking up at 4:30 and decided to stay in bed. At 4:55, I thought about just getting up and starting my day, but I forced myself to stay in bed a little longer, until about 5:15. I normally get up at 6 a.m.

I got up and went downstairs to start my day with my standard routine of reading and coffee. I'm 39 now, and I started drinking coffee for the first time about two years ago. I read a book about Starbucks by its founder and was fascinated by his description of the coffee and his business. So I decided to give it a go. I now enjoy drinking a cup of coffee or two a day.

This morning I went to Yarrow, and it was a great testing session. The sessions seem to make me happy. I feel like I'm making progress. I had Julian and Matt over for this one. Julian was setting up his grill for cooking, so I briefed Matt on an event I wanted him to test.

**5 ROUNDS OF:**

**RUN 400 METERS**

**10 CLEANS OVER THE HAY BALES PLUS BURPEES OVER THE BALES**

I had three hay bales stacked up for a total height of 40 inches. I wanted to see if the hay would be stable or compress. Generally speaking, I just wanted to see what would happen to the hay. Also, I wanted to see the effects of the combo in that test. I don't think we have ever had the athletes clean an object over a wall and then do a burpee over the wall. We for sure have done burpees over a wall and burpees over an object. This year in Event 6 at Regionals, the individuals did burpees over the box and then cleans. Now we are combining the two. When I told Matt the weight was 100 lb., he said, "*Oh, we are using the women's weight.*"

"*Trust me,*" I said. "*It's going to bite.*"

I want this one to force athletes to just push, and I don't want them to have to slow up—unless they get gassed.

Before starting the test, Matt and I discussed what he thought his time should be. He said he was shooting for 15 minutes. I said 17-18. He laughed and said OK, but he said he would push for 15.

Matt did his first run in 1:45 and finished his first round in 3:13.

His second round was finished at 6:57, for a round time of 3:44. I saw it was going to be gassier and more challenging than expected.

He finished Round 3 at 10:56, around 4 minutes for that round.

On Round 4 he started slowing up on the burpee section, and that round was finished at 14:49, around 3:53 for the round.

His final round was strong. He finished everything at 18:13, making that round 3:24. He had pushed his pace on the final piece a lot harder and ended up with a final round that was faster than all other rounds but the first.

Matt was gassed, and he really liked the test. I liked it, too. I can see this one going down to the wire with an incredible race. Julian expressed interest in trying this one, and I told him *"not today."* I had seen what I needed to see. I might have him try it another time.

Later, Matt made a comment about my nailing the time.

*"I guess you know what you are doing,"* he said.

Yeah, I kinda do.

After that, we had Julian test the sledgehammer/Assault-bike event, which might be Saturday night's test. I had him do this:

### 30 CALORIES ON THE ASSAULT BIKE

### 20 FEET ON THE BANGER

We only had a 10-foot metal lane for the Banger, so we had him do 10 feet down and 10 back. It's such a simple sprint test. Moments before he started, I told him to redline it. He nodded in agreement, and then Stephane started the clock.

Julian finished the 30 calories in 37 seconds, which is insane; I think I recently did 30 calories in 2 minutes.

He then started crushing the Banger and finished 10 feet at the 1:50 mark, so he did 10 feet in roughly a minute. Let's say it took him 13 seconds of transition time. This is something I should have noted, but I was distracted and didn't.

At the 10-foot mark, he turned around and came back to finish at 3:01. The second 10 feet were slightly slower than the first 10.

Julian went to the ground after wobbling away from the implement, and I asked him how it felt. He said it hurt. It looked like it hurt. I might have Matt test this to see what a smaller guy gets. Three minutes is right in the time domain I want for this one. It's a sprint, an all-out effort. I texted Bill and said, "*Let's go with the 20-foot lane.*" What's hilarious is that I was originally thinking 50 feet, which would have taken a long time. This is why we test these things—especially the ones with odd objects rarely seen in typical CrossFit training.

Reluctantly, I might not get any programming in for the next two days while traveling, so I might not make any entries. Maybe I can squeeze some quick sessions in and just take a look at everything.

*Thursday, June 15, 3:02 p.m.*
I was able to leave Santa Cruz yesterday evening, which really made me happy. Our meetings were originally supposed to go until today, but some stuff came up and we were able to finish everything yesterday. Having our own plane makes it convenient to leave and get home fast from Santa Cruz. The plane ride isn't incredibly fast, but avoiding the drive to the airport, security and all that makes the trip faster. The range on the plane is also limiting. It's great for small trips but nothing really beyond California or Arizona.

I went into Yarrow earlier today and looked at the schedule. Today is not a test day. I might not test tomorrow either. I haven't decided yet. I contemplated moving 17.5++ to Sunday again, and I actually made the switch. But I really like it as a Saturday-night event, so I moved it back. I'm still undecided on where it will end up. With the big squat in the thruster, Saturday is actually a good time to do it. As of right now, Saturday is relatively light on the legs in terms of squatting. Yes, they have some heavy squat cleans, but just a few. These guys and gals are completely capable of handling some heavy squat cleans and then heavy thrusters hours later. I don't like that both the thruster and clean events are in a similar time domain. I'll continue to look at it.

Speaking of the clean test, I thought of changing it up a little. After seeing Julian do it, I think it's a little longer than I want. I'm thinking 8 regular pull-ups instead of 8 chest-to-bars, then the squat cleans. But as I thought about it more, I ended up considering 4 bar muscle-ups. There are a few reasons I like this. It's more dramatic with the full-body movement and large range of motion—much more exciting than toes-to-bars and pull-ups. There is also a small opportunity for people to fail muscle-ups even though the reps are low and they shouldn't. Four bar muscle-ups will also be faster than 8 chest-to-bar pull-ups and 8 toes-to-bars. They'll probably even be faster than 8 regular pull-ups and 8 toes-to-bars.

I also really like its clean presentation: 8 rounds of 4 bar muscle-ups and 2 cleans (*ascending weight*). Although it's small and silly, it means a lot to me that 4 muscle-up reps multiplied by 2 cleans equals 8—the number of rounds. So the numbers play well with each other.

I want to test this version, and I need to find a stronger CrossFit athlete for that. I've reached out to a few, and I'm waiting to hear back.

Oh yeah—yesterday while I was gone we received a shipment of weights to make heavier Worms. I'm going to reach out to one of the Orange County teams that finished outside the top five to ask if the members will test some events for me. But I really haven't worked on Team events yet, so that will have to wait.

*7:34 p.m.*

Spent some time in Yarrow today trying to figure out some Sunday events. Most of today, even when I've been away from Yarrow, I've been thinking about Sunday and possible finale and pre-finale events.

At various stages of the season—Open, Regionals, Games—I often have tough phases in which I can't make a breakthrough, and then all of a sudden something clicks and it all falls together. Those are some of my most joyous programming moments, especially during the Open.

As I was walking out of my house to go to Yarrow, I had a thought that I just keep focusing on. It's about the interval event I had toyed with before. Once I got to Yarrow, I started sketching out some ideas.

The general idea was 2 minutes of work, rest 1 minute, repeat 3 times. The first two movements would be fixed work, like 10 HSPU and 15 calories, and then the third thing would be heavy deadlifts—I haven't decided on a movement here. So you would do the HSPU and the calories, and then with the remaining time you would do as many deadlifts as you could, advancing the load down the floor. At the beginning of Rounds 2 and 3, someone could have the bar further down the floor than other athletes. Ideally, I could select a total number of deadlift reps that would allow them to finish in Round 3.

Let's say over the course of the 3 rounds it's 50 deadlifts total. In Round 1 an athlete gets 15, and in Round 2 he gets 21, so he'd have to do 14 in Round 3 to finish the event. Others might have to do 10 or 20. I like this conceptually, but it will take a lot of testing to get the timing, movements and loading right. That said, I'm not set on this format yet.

I then considered another idea I had early on in the process: HSPU, row and then something that covers distance, like a handstand walk, a pull or lunges. So maybe this becomes three short sprint events. I like these kinds of events because it's very exciting whenever people race down the floor. I need to decide if the sections all tie to each other or if they're scored separately. Maybe even two separate scored events. I like that idea more than 3 events. It could be two separate scored events with a 2-minute rest in between. If I did that, I would almost want the events to be different. If they are scored separately, I feel like they should test different things.

Plenty to think about tomorrow and work with, but I feel like I'm making some progress now. No testing tomorrow. That will help the ideation process of putting events to paper.

We also received word today that Christian Lucero passed his secondary test, which means his Regional testing is over and clean. I'm surprised. The way he handled that situation and his actions led me to believe he was guilty. But maybe he cycled off in time to avoid being caught by the tests. This is a thought of mine, but he passed the test, so that thought is not backed by evidence, just suspicion.

*Friday, June 16, 1:18 p.m.*
I'm still trying to figure out the Sunday finale. I spent a few hours at Yarrow playing with ideas. I was able to sketch out a few options. Not really feeling any of them. But most include HSPU and now rope climbs. I also had one idea of including the Assault AirRunner. I haven't ever programmed a runner like that at the Games because of the ease of running outside. But it would be an interesting twist to include it. I would use a short distance. Like 100s. Still going to play with this and process some ideas.

*Saturday, June 17, 10:48 a.m.*

Yesterday was a really bad day for me and programming. As you can tell by my entry, I didn't get much done and didn't have much enthusiasm for the process or the day. I tried hard. I spent some time at Yarrow trying to be creative, but it wasn't happening. I even took a nap on the floor there thinking I would wake up refreshed and ready. I didn't. I actually went home and did some CrossFit work, then ended up napping again. I think yesterday was just a bad day for me physically and mentally.

Today I'm ready to go. I feel good. I've been thinking a lot about the teams. I decided to step away from the individuals today to get some events done for the teams. I think it will help me get past a mental block I'm having with the Individual competition, particularly Sunday.

Some of the Team ideas I have include a row and the Worm—a row/Worm couplet. Something like row 30 calories (*25 for women*) and then Worm work, 4-6 rounds for time. But the cool twist is each team will have six rowers, so everybody works at the same time. Sixty rowers on the floor. This is something we could never do at Regionals, but the Games is the place for crazy stuff.

Another idea I have is to do the final event with 50 clean and jerks again—but with the heavy Worm. Remember, I had Bill create a couple of extra Worms, so now we have the standard Worm and options for lighter and heavier Worms. Bill sent me a bunch of fillers, so I'm going to play with those combos this weekend. We're coordinating a team to come and test next Saturday.

The current Worm is 435 lb. The lighter Worm will have loads of 65 lb. for men and 55 lb. for women—390 lb. total. The heavier Worm will either weigh 555 or 510 lb. I have to play with those options and see what I want to use. I need to see how heavy 555 really is. Bill mentioned something I'm worried about: hitting people on the head. We had a few people tweak their necks and hit themselves in the head at Regionals. So to get away from that, I won't have them take the heavy Worms over the head. Worm deadlift, Worm clean to shoulder, drop. Worm front squat. Stuff like that.

*12:03 p.m.*

I had a good session today on the Team stuff.

I worked on the Saturday schedule. I feel Thursday is close to being set. Team Run-Swim-Run and then Team Amanda. The first event is a pairs test. The second is individual efforts for a combined score.

Friday is close to set. O-course to start the day. Some sort of Worm and row test (*as of right now*), and a snatch event.

For Saturday, I want to do the same clean ladder the individuals are doing but formatted for teams. I was thinking about using a format like we used in Regionals two years ago, where all three members snatched. To do this, I had to make some changes to the schedule. Basically, all Team men will go in 4 heats, then the women will go. So it will be split competitions for the teams for that event.

I then played with a Saturday-morning north-lot event. I'm thinking some sort of team clean and run, but I'm worried about having 20 teams going at the same time, which is what I have now. I need to play with this a little more. But I'm making progress, and that feels good.

*6:39 p.m.*
Spent some time at Yarrow tonight working on the Team stuff. Didn't make a ton of progress on actual events, but I did lay everything out in a separate room just for teams. I need the visuals separate. The Individual and Team competitions need to speak to each other and play off each other, but I also need to see them as individual units.

I also listed all the 2017 Regional workout movements to compare what we did there with what I'm doing here. At the Games, they will touch the barbell, but at Regionals they did not. I was planning on leaning on the Worm a lot again, but I might not.

I plan on meeting with Stephane tomorrow and going over all the Age Group events. I haven't really looked at those yet, but they want my signoff on them, and it would be good to have those in place early.

Our meeting in Madison is in about 10 days. I'll have a lot done by then, but not all of it. I feel OK with where I'm at. Not enthusiastic. But I'm making progress. I just need to keep getting in here.

Oh, and I'm watching some of the U.S. Open this weekend. It's a great tournament and competition so far.

*Sunday, June 18, 12:19 p.m.*

Today I met with Stephane to go over the Age Group programming he and Pat created. They did a good job on the first round. I had some feedback for them, and they will now go back and make a round of edits before presenting the programming to me again in a few days.

I gave them a few notes. I did not like their inclusion of 100% from the Games last year. The event was 40 box jumps and 20 D-ball cleans. During that event, we had one athlete, Alethea Boon, blow out her Achilles. The event for the individuals was fine, but for 120 athletes in the 35-39, 40-44 and 45-49 divisions, I think it might be pushing our luck. The last thing we need is more injuries from certain movements, like the box jump. We didn't anticipate the ring-dip issue at Regionals. I contend that nobody did. But the box jump, in this workout, in this format, it's best not to include it at all.

They included a 1RM snatch for the teens and the younger Age Group block (35-39, 40-44, 45-49). For the advanced age group (50-54, 55-59, 60+), they are doing a 2RM front squat instead. They had a lot of Olympic-type movements across a lot of workouts, so I offered some ways to reduce the number. But overall it looks good, and it's going in the right direction. It will be good to get these locked in, especially with the new format that has the Age Group events running at the same time as other parts of the competition.

*12:44 p.m.*

I decided to go back to the Sunday events for the individuals and just start sketching some ideas down on a pad of paper. Sometimes I need to do that—just write, see what happens. I don't want to say I made a breakthrough, but I made some serious progress. I sketched out a couple of options for events I want to test.

First was the interval idea. I want to use that as an event, so I wrote down some ideas for testing. I decided to start with 1-2 rope climbs. The final number will depend on how long it takes to climb the higher rig Bill is making for me. Then row 20 calories, or less, depending on timing. And then X split snatches, alternating legs each round. Finish the rope climbs and the calories, then do as many split snatches as possible in the remainder of the 2-minute window. Then rest 1 minute. Repeat that 3-4 times.

In the final round, you do whatever's left of the total number of reps. For example, the total number might be 75. If you did 70 in the first few rounds, you would have 5 left. Someone else might have only done 60 reps, so he would have 15 left. I would figure out the total number in testing.

I'm actually feeling this concept play out, and I think it can make for an exciting event with an exciting finish. This would not be the final but the pre-final. I like it.

I worked on the final next. I want to hit some handstand push-ups, probably with a deficit. Maybe an escalating deficit—each round the deficit increases, and perhaps it decreases, too. Do a set, do some other stuff, and then come back. Last year we had HSPU on the rings, and the year before we had one set of HSPU on the wall in Pedal to the Metal 2. Last year, I wasn't really happy with how things played out—especially the judging and the standards, which were inconsistent on the rings. I want to take a break from that movement, which is usually not my style. Typically, I would come back just to make sure we got it right, but this time I'm going to step away from it for a year at least.

For this one, I was thinking 10-15 HSPU and 10-14 weighted pistols for 3 rounds. On each round, the HSPU get deeper and the pistol weight gets heavier, probably with kettlebells. Then it ends with a long lunge down the floor with two kettlebells. Or two dumbbells. The lunging finishes always play out well.

Between these tests, I like what we're starting to see. In the first one we have a large upper-body pull—I might even make it a legless climb—then a large leg-dependent pull on the rower. The snatch is a nice technical full-body movement. All this comes in interval style, which we typically don't do at the Games. Lots of athletes train this way now, but we don't test it that often.

In the second event, the final, I like the upper-body push (*I will allow kipping*), the single-leg squat, and the finish with the full-body work required by overhead walking lunges. These movements not only play well with each other in the event but also sing nicely to the other tests that day.

Something else helped me get here: I'm taking the handstand walk completely out of the afternoon events. I'm thinking about adding it to the work test Sunday morning. So it would be like this: Move three objects down the field, but each time you come across the field, you have to use a handstand walk. That could get nasty, but it balances out that event—

meaning it's not just a strongman test. It's a strongman-like test with a lot of gymnastics involved.

I'm happy with today's progress. It's Sunday and Father's Day, and I feel like I was given a nice present today: progress on programming the Sunday finale of the CrossFit Games.

*6:30 p.m.*
I just made a quick hour-long trip to Yarrow, and I butchered the Saturday and Sunday schedules.

As I was sitting around the house today after leaving Yarrow earlier, I was watching golf, reading, working on my motorcycle and thinking about the schedule. The progress I made earlier today on the final two events for Sunday gave me confidence in a format I want to use for those blocks.

So looking at Sunday, I had some strongman-like moves on the field, with a handstand walk. Then a rope-climb/row/weightlifting interval workout. Then a final that involves HSPU, pistols and lunges. My problem with Saturday continues to be the test with the med-ball clean followed by the test with the barbell clean. It's a small detail, but it's huge to me.

After seeing what I came up with for Sunday, it dawned on me that a switch could make sense.

So now I'm moving the run/hay-bale event from Saturday to Sunday morning and putting the strongman event on Saturday in the run/hay spot. Of course, this has a huge ripple effect. I had to take a look at the schedule and see how I can do this and still preserve the noon-1 p.m. live window we have on CBS. That window has been a pain in my ass with this whole schedule, but it's the nature of the beast when working with major TV networks.

This change means the Team workouts on Saturday and Sunday morning will likely be different now, and it also means hay bales will not be on the floor for the other divisions like I thought they would be.

I texted Stephane once I made this decision and told him not to do the exact Individual run/hay-bale test for the age groups. That was something I had suggested earlier, but now it doesn't make sense. I feel better about the schedule even though I made major changes to it today.

On Saturday, individuals will do strongman-like moves with some handstand walks in their first event. Then they'll do bar muscle-ups with low reps of very heavy squat cleans in their second. Finally, they'll do some double-unders with heavy thrusters for high reps. Those all play well together and complement each other. I'm aware of the repetitive nature of the squatting in the clean and the thruster, but in terms of their physical demands, they are very different movements. If the squat-clean workout were lighter and contained more reps, then high-rep heavy thrusters would not play well later. But Saturday is shaping up nicely now.

On Sunday, it's looking like run/clean/burpee for the first event, then rope climbs/row/barbell—probably deadlift, sumo deadlift, maybe split snatch—on the next. Finally, we'll end with some handstand push-ups, pistols and lunges. So it won't be too squatty. The pistols will provide some squatting, but they won't be so bad. We'll end with a horrifically hard lunge walk. This new schedule also takes the handstand walk and the handstand push-ups off the same day.

Tomorrow is another testing day with Julian. I'm going to have him test the new version of the pull-up/toes-to-bars/clean ladder. Instead of pull-ups and toes-to-bars, I'm going to make it just bar muscle-ups. I discussed at length with Stephane the weight of the bars based off the athletes' reported 1RMs. Basically, it appears that a quarter of the field might complete it if we end at 365 lb. I think I want to see more than that complete it, so we're going to drop it down to 350. The numbers we've collected suggest around half should finish it then. That makes more sense. We'll get a sense of what it feels like and how it looks tomorrow when we have Julian test it.

*Monday, June 19, 6:57 p.m.*
Julian was sick today, so we didn't test, but I ended up doing a lot of work on the Games, mostly schedule tweaks and refinement. I had a call with Joe Novello, our TV-production expert, and Justin to discuss the schedule and the broadcast teams. The call went well, and it made me realize I needed to do a once-over on the schedule for the O-course and snatch events for the teams and individuals. I went through them once more and then shared them with the team so they have an idea of what we're doing in those blocks.

I also changed the snatch event for the individuals: They're going to lift on their own now. My first version had them lifting two at a time, but the change will make it easier to cover and tell a better story. But if we make that change, the athletes only get two lifts. So every Individual athlete will get two lifts, and then the top 10 lifters will advance to get an additional two lifts. For the teams, I committed to doing it in a 20-minute heat. Each heat of 14 *(or 13)* teams will have 7 minutes for all males to establish 1RMs. We'll have a 1-minute transition, and then the women of the teams will have 7 minutes to establish 1RM snatches.

With Stephane, I also looked over some of the Age Group programming that he and Pat had changed. I like it. I had some more feedback, but it's close.

We're going to test tomorrow—with Julian or not. If he can't show up, we'll have Matt test. Actually, maybe I'll have them both test the bar-muscle-up/clean workout at the same time.

*Wednesday, June 20, 4:14 p.m.*
I had a couple of good sessions at Yarrow today. I met Stephane and Matt there. Julian couldn't make it. I had Matt warm up while I worked on the schedule and Stephane worked on the Age Group events.

For the schedule, I worked on Saturday and dug into what should happen. I also committed to having the teams snatch on Friday and really hashed out how it will go down. Joe needed some extra time between the start of Saturday's Team events and the break in the Individual events, so I created that. I also committed to a Big Bob event on Saturday morning for the teams. It will probably be a Big Bob race for distance, but I haven't decided yet. Truthfully, that event probably won't be determined until the week of the Games. I don't have a Big Bob here, and I don't know how the surface will affect the sled. Bill is also reducing the width of the Big Bob for us, and I imagine that will make it a tad lighter. With all that in mind, the Big Bob event will just be a placeholder until we can fully test it at the Games.

Once Matt was ready, I had him do a simple test on the concept of Sunday's final. I say concept because, as I told Matt, things will probably change 10 times before we determine the actual event. But I wanted some baseline info. I had him do this:

3 ROUNDS OF:

10 PARALLETTE HANDSTAND PUSH-UPS

10 PISTOLS WITH A 45-LB. DUMBBELL

I had him do the 10 HSPU strict, and the first round took him 54 seconds total.

For the second round, I had him switch to kipping HSPU. It took a brief moment for him to set the distance of the parallettes from the wall and get his kip in sync. He eventually finished the second round at 2:50.

In Round 3 he was doing the HSPU in twos and threes. He finished 3 rounds in 5:09.

I want to add lunges to the end of this, so that was too long. I would like to have it tested again after tweaking the reps and weight. Matt mentioned that holding the dumbbell in the front rack position really taxed his arms for the HSPU. That's interesting. I'll also test it again with kipping HSPU throughout. I want to keep this portion of the test in the 2:30-3:30 range, so I need to get the time down. I think he could probably do it again in 4:00 if he were allowed to kip the entire time. I would also like to test with a higher-level athlete—not just yet but once I narrow it down a little.

On that note, I decided to have some of our Demo Team members out to test in a week or two, right after our upcoming Madison meeting. Julian is working out great, but he's local, which means he comes down and then drives home the same day. When I had Dan Bailey here last year, or Brooke Ence, I was able to test, take a break and then retest again later in the day. With Dan I did this multiple times throughout the day. I need that availability again.

I need some women to test, too, so I told Stephane to email Alex Parker and Kelley Jackson to see if they could come out for three days of testing. Kelley is important because she's a smaller female, and I want to see how the 70-lb. dumbbell will affect her on the GHD event. I also asked him to get Paul Tremblay to come out. Graham Holmberg is also on the team, and today I asked Ben Alderman to join. Two years ago, Ben asked me how he could make it onto the team, and I said, *"Place higher at Regionals."* This year he placed 11th, and I like him, so he got an invitation.

This evening I came back and focused on the Team programming. I have a team coming on Saturday to test, so I need to get some stuff done for them.

I played around with what I want the teams to do at different stages, I looked at what they're already doing, and I laid out the known events.

The first day has a pairs relay with little true teamwork: the Run-Swim-Run. The second event on that first day uses individual efforts that sum to a team score. So no true teamwork. That's the Team Amanda event. I also realized today that I don't want to call it Team Amanda.

On Friday, the first event is again a relay involving individual efforts: the O-course. The second event on Friday is another that uses the sum of individual efforts: the 1RM snatch. So the first three events are really devoid of teamwork. This is fine at this stage because these are important tests and good events. But that means Friday night's event must involve a lot of teamwork. And that leads me to the Worm. So I worked on that.

I'm thinking I'll have all six members row 30/25 calories then perform 21 Worm cleans. In the next round, they'll row the same calories but do 15 cleans. In the final round, we'll use the same row calories and 9 cleans. We might use one of the new Worms. We're going to test those implements this weekend, and we now have three different loads. The heavy Worm will be really heavy, so I need to experiment and see what's possible with it.

Saturday morning has a Big Bob event in which all six athletes work together. Saturday midday is not created yet, but I now know a few things about it. I'll probably have them work either as pairs or trios. It will be more traditional, with a barbell and some normal CrossFit elements—probably relay style with a lot of teamwork. Saturday night will end with a team Worm event—maybe bar muscle-ups and Worm something.

Sunday morning, it's looking like they'll use the 400-meter run course. Originally, I was thinking they would run with the litter or something like that. But the more I play it out, I really don't know if I want to use the litter again. It didn't generate the stimulus I needed when we used it before, and it probably won't over 400 meters. But I did come to this: Maybe I'll have them run the 400 with a Worm—possibly the light Worm—then return and do some paired burpee box jumps over the hay bales. This might be a second event I'll have the team test on Saturday.

Really, it will be about testing the Worm run. I don't remember if we have ever had them run with the Worm at the Games. But this might be the year to do that.

For the Sunday final, I came up with something like this: clean, squat, drop, step over, repeat—with the heavy Worm. That will be annoying as hell and require a lot of team coordination. And it's probably something they haven't practiced. I might want to pair that with rope climbs because that setup will be on the floor. The big twist: The team must hold another Worm as one person runs over to the rope, climbs, comes back and tags someone out. I just thought of something else: We can combine that with the HSPU wall. So maybe four people hold the Worm while two work. OK, lots of progress and potential here. I'm going to have fun with this one.

Today when I was working with Stephane and Matt, I had a bunch of things going on and my mind was not focused. Matt asked me a question, and I said, "Hold on. I am all over the place. I need to focus." I took a moment and just thought about the one thing I needed to do at that moment, and it helped ground me. It's interesting because that feeling, what was going on for me, comes from a good place. I feel good with where I am right now in this whole process. The Games are coming along great, and in my mind they are going to be the best version yet. I feel confident in that, and I feel good right now. I just need to keep making consistent progress and continue this flow, and I'll be in a great head space leading into the Games. As of now, I'm in a great head space going into our Madison meeting next week.

*Wednesday, June 21, 4:19 p.m.*
This morning we tested with Matt. We got some new dead-blow sledge-hammers that are about a pound and a half heavier than the ones we had.

We had him test this:

### 30 CALORIES ON THE ASSAULT BIKE

### 20 FEET OF STRIKING

Matt started off slower on the bike than Julian and was off at just over a minute.

Once he started his swings, things seemed fine, but soon it was not looking good. He had to take a couple of breaks to rest.

Matt ended up finishing in just over 4 minutes. Julian had done it in about 3 minutes. Matt stated that his grip was wrecked. We then compared the two hammers and found the new one was about 6 inches longer. That actually took some of the power from the swing in the setup we had. I took a few swings at it and found the taller handle bunched you up so you couldn't generate a powerful swing. We found another place that makes and sells hammers, and we ordered more shorter ones. The first hammers we had used featured the company's name engraved into aggressive knurling, and the handles ate our hands up.

Stephane and I also reviewed the Masters events some more. I like where they're ending up, but I gave some feedback that will improve them—mainly around time domains. A handful of events seemed to be in the same time domain, so I suggested making one longer. As is, the only longer event they have is the Run-Swim-Run. I think they need a longer CrossFit event, too. We worked on that.

This afternoon I cleaned up more schedule items and made some progress on finalizing Saturday. Stephane showed me the layout if we did heats of 20 for the Banger, and it was really tight, so we decided to do heats of 14-13-13. But that change means I must add two heats to the schedule. Once I had added the heats, I had to massage and manage the schedule in other places.

I also worked on the Team events. I have a pretty good idea of all of the events I want to do—minus one test. I put down some notes and possibilities for that undetermined event. It will be a more traditional Team event in that it will have barbells, GHDs, pull-ups and stuff like that. But I want it to be unique, so I might have them start in pairs, then finish in trios. Not sure yet. Playing with some ideas. But it will be good.

My Yarrow neighbor is a pain in the ass. Shortly after I moved in, he walked through my gym, into my office and said, "*Who is the guy who comes here on the motorcycle and plays the music really loud?*" I told him it was me and asked him if he thought this little speaker was too loud. His intrusion into my space and complaint about the "*guy on the motorcycle*" started our relationship on a bad track, and since then it's only become worse. He of course complains when we drop barbells. The other day he complained about Julian's use of his Traeger to cook food, and yesterday he left a note on our door complaining about the hay remnants that are around our gym and outside.

Today he had the nerve to come over and complain about the hay to me, and I was very short with him. He threatened to take pictures and tell the landlord. I told him, "*Please do.*" I also told him it seems everything we do is a problem and all he does is complain.

I can't stand the guy. As great as this place is for me, I'll be so happy when I move up north and have a new testing facility.

*Thursday, June 22, 2:25 p.m.*

This morning we tested at 10 a.m. Julian was able to show up today, so I had him test the new version of the clean ladder. Last time he tested the version that had 8 pull-ups and 8 toes-to-bars with ascending cleans up to 365. For this version, I reduced the loads. And I changed the body-weight movement to bar muscle-ups.

8 ROUNDS OF:

4 MUSCLE-UPS

2 CLEANS (225, 245, 265, 285, 305, 320, 335, 350 LB.)

His first round was fast—30 seconds.

His second round was complete at 1:34.

At 2:45, he was done with this third round.

His fourth ended at 3:58. He had started to take breaks between his cleans. He never broke up his muscle-ups, but the rest between cleans got longer and longer.

He finished the 6th round—with cleans at 320 lb.—at 5:17.

Round 7 was finished at 7:06.

Now it was time for the big bar, the 350. Last time we tested, he did 2 at 345 but zero at 365. At 8:37, he set up and went for the lift but missed. He paced around and took a bit of a breather before giving the bar another legit attempt. On the second attempt, he snuck under the weight, hung out for a minute and then stood up at the 9:36 mark. I waved him off and said, "*Good.*" We all agreed a 10-minute cap would be perfect here. I was impressed by his performance, and I was happy with how it played out. I like this version much better. It's quicker, and that's what I'm looking for. I think the best guys will finish in the mid-to-high fives.

Next, I had him do 20 split snatches for time with the 100-lb. dumbbell. He predicted it would take him just under a minute. I said it would take longer. He did it in 1:10. I was impressed. We had Matt do it, too. It took him

1:50. I don't know if I'm going to do anything with that or what I want the data for, but it's good to have the numbers in the back pocket.

This afternoon I went back to Yarrow and worked on the schedule, refining some times and solidifying some points. I'm feeling good about where I am today.

Big testing day this weekend with the team. Experimenting with the new Worms.

Then off to Madison on Monday.

*Friday, June 23, 12:52 p.m.*
I was moving in a lot of directions this morning.

Our community pool is putting in a hot tub, and we were told yesterday that it would be done today. The girls wanted to go check it out even though the marine layer was still upon us. When we got there, we saw it was still closed. But we got into the pool anyway and played around. I was so distracted. I could only think about the testing and what I wanted Julian to do later in the morning. Normally I can shelve distractions and focus on what I need to do, but at this stage it's hard not to think about testing.

I arrived to Yarrow a little late because of another call I had to do. Once there, we warmed up with some basketball, and then I let Julian know what I wanted to test: 15-12-9 kettlebell deadlifts with the 200s and handstand push-ups on parallettes. After discussing the reps and loading, as well as the time domain I was looking to hit, I decided to drop the reps to 12-9-6. At the 2015 Games we used a similar deadlift weight and had them do 8 reps total. So 15-12-9 would be significantly more, but even 12-9-6 is a lot more. I decided to start with the HSPU, not the deads.

12-9-6 REPS OF:

PARALLETTE HSPU

KETTLEBELL DEADLIFTS (200 LB.)

Julian's first round was blazing fast. The 12 handstand push-ups were completed in 21 seconds, and his 12 deadlifts were done at 58 seconds. He broke the deadlifts into 2 sets.

His set of 9 HSPU was again unbroken and complete at 1:22. His 9 deadlifts were complete at 2:11, also broken into 2 sets.

For his final set of 6 handstand push-ups, he kicked up but lost his balance, then kicked back up and completed the set. On his final 6 deadlifts, he did 4, put the kettlebells down, then finished the last 2 at 2:52.

Once he finished the set of 9 at 2:11, I realized this was going to be very fast, so I went and found a 70-lb. kettlebell and placed it on the floor as he was finishing his final round. As soon as he finished, I told him to take the kettlebell overhead and lunge it 80 feet. He regained his composure a little and without complaining started lunging with the kettlebell at 3:17. He lunged 40 feet, put it down, turned around and returned. He finished that effort at 4:27.

The loading is not right on the lunge. I will probably use two objects overhead, but the stimulus and the visual are there. I like where this one is going. I have some changes I might want to make but need to think it through more.

One thought I just had about this test: We don't have an ascending-reps test in the Games yet—an event that starts with a low number of reps and then climbs. Maybe flipping this one will be good.

After a brief period of rest, I asked Julian to test this:

IN 2 MINUTES:

I LEGLESS ROPE CLIMB (20 FEET)

20 CALORIES ON THE CONCEPT2

AS MANY WEIGHTED PISTOLS AS POSSIBLE IN REMAINING TIME

He did the climb up and down in 9 seconds.

He finished 20 calories at 1:05.

With 55 seconds remaining, he was able to get 19 weighted pistols. This test would involve a 1-minute break, and we'd repeat it 3-4 times.

I told him he had 30 seconds before he was going to do it again. As he started the rope climb, I decided to change the last movement. The pistols just don't look good there. They're fine in training, sure, but for an event like this at the CrossFit Games, no. I had Matt set up a bar with 135 lb. by the time Julian was on the rower. Julian finished the rope climb and the row at 1:24, and I told him to do as many OHS as possible in the remaining time. He got 11.

That was all I had him do. I like where this one is going, but it needs more refining. I think I might make it two trips up and down the rope and reduce the calories on the rower. As I started playing that out, I thought about just ditching the rower entirely. Logistically, it's hard to get in and out of the rower. And in a 2-minute time frame, those seconds add up fast. So I might just pull the SkiErg from the GHD event and put the rower there. I think the GHD/row/push-press combo will still be a great core stinger and a great event to get the heart rate going. If I move the SkiErg to the interval event, athletes just walk over and start pulling hard on the SkiErg instead of strapping in.

After we wrapped up, I went home, grabbed some lunch and came back to meet with Stephane about the Age Group programming. I just made some small suggestions for changes, but the events are very close. For the past hour or so, I've been taking a dive into the Individual stuff again. One thing I'm noticing is I that don't have a really long test. The Run-Swim-Run is probably the longest, but I'm assuming it's around 30 minutes—probably 25 for the fastest. In last year's Games, I think I had at least two events that were over 30 minutes—the long run and the Murph version.

I need to process this and think about it.

*Saturday, June 24, 2:32 p.m.*
Very large day of programming and planning.

I showed up at Yarrow at 7 a.m. to do the CrossFit.com WOD with an old Army friend of mine. It was a very long workout: as many rounds as possible in 45 minutes of run 800 meters, 10 deadlifts at 315 lb., run 800 meters, 50 sit-ups. My friend, Ben, is still on active duty in one of those roles I can't talk about, but we go way back. When I was first stationed in DLI in Monterey, he was a young Army private learning Spanish, and I was in my first year or so of CrossFit. He was athletic and strong, and he had played college football. We started training together, and a great friendship was born from that. We followed CrossFit.com religiously back then, so it was a nice reunion to do today's workout together.

Shortly after we finished, Julian showed up. I had him test the event with the running, hay-bale cleans and burpees. Matt had already done it, but I wanted to test it again with a slightly longer run and 9 reps instead of 10. The odd number will have athletes land on the side nearest the finish line, so it's a natural choice.

I had Julian run 500 meters. Matt's run was closer to 400.

**5 ROUNDS OF:**

**RUN 500 METERS**

**9 CLEANS OVER THE HAY BALES PLUS BURPEES OVER THE BALES**

Round 1 went smoothly. He did the run in 2:14 and finished the entire round by 3:27.

Round 2 was finished at 7:03.

Julian kept near that pace for most of the workout. He finished Round 3 at 10:45 and Round 4 at 14:50.

All 5 rounds were complete at 18:30.

This was slightly longer than Matt's test, but Matt had a shorter run and 1 additional rep each round. I want to ensure the test will be closer to 20 minutes rather than 15. I think the version Matt did will be about 16-17. This version with the longer run will hit that 18-minute mark. I still might tweak the reps to make it longer. Each round of 9 cleans and burpees over the hay took roughly 1 minute. So if I wanted to add 30 seconds per round, I could add 3-5 reps to get a time closer to 20:30 or so. I might do that. Make it run 500 meters, 15 hay-bale cleans and burpees, 5 rounds. If I decide to make that change, I'll test it again before committing.

I had planned it so a team showed up as soon as Julian finished but wouldn't see what he was doing. I don't like crossing over workouts with testers. Just because you test an event—or even two or four—doesn't mean you get access to what everyone is doing. For the most part, I try to keep the testers and testing separate.

The team was CrossFit Forest, which finished 10th at the California Regional. First, I had them play around with the new Worms. I had them do some cleans and front squats, and then some thrusters. They progressed with few issues. The heavy Worm was obviously heavy for them, but they were still able to cycle it.

After they played around with the Worm, I asked them to test a workout. I really only had the row/squat concept at the time, but on the spot I came up with the actual reps. I told them I would like each member to row 40/30 cals at the same time, and then they'd do 21-15-9 front squats with the Worm. Having seen them do reps with the heavy Worm earlier, I decided to change the reps to 30-20-10 while they were talking strategy.

As we talked about the rowing, I wondered if I should drop the female calories—40/25 or something like that. We decided just to do it as originally written.

ROW 40/30 CALORIES AT THE SAME TIME

30 FRONT SQUATS WITH THE WORM

ROW 40/30 CALORIES AT THE SAME TIME

20 FRONT SQUATS WITH THE WORM

ROW 40/30 CALORIES AT THE SAME TIME

I0 FRONT SQUATS WITH THE WORM

The first male finished his 40 in 1:27, and the whole team was done by 1:37. So the 40/30 split was pretty much spot on. I was pleased with that. They did the 30 squats with the heavy Worm unbroken in 1:13, finishing the first round at 3:13.

On the second round, the row took closer to 2 minutes for some and over 2 minutes for others. The variance between first and last was about 22 seconds. Interestingly, one of the females, Kendall Morris, finished first. She crushed it. She ended up being the all-star for the team in terms of attitude, effort and pure ability that day. I was impressed with her. The second set of squats took about 50 seconds, and they were unbroken. Total time after 2 rounds: 6:57.

On the final round of rowing, they all started at roughly 7:15, and Kendall was off first at 8:55. The last person, a small female, was off at 9:42. This round generated the most variance on the row, and that was to be expected because it was the final round after a ton of work. It took them 55 seconds to finish the last round of squats for a total time of 10:55.

As I think about this one, I think the 40/30 split is good, but I might increase the reps a little on the squats, maybe do 30/25/20. I also went into the schedule and looked at how much time I have for this event on Friday. It was a 12-minute window, but I adjusted it to 15 so I have more time for a stiff test. This will be the only true CrossFit work they do on Friday, so I need to make it stick. Earlier in the day, they do the O-course and the 1RM snatch.

Next, I had the team test some running with the Worm. I told them to pick it up and run 2 laps around my building, basically 500 meters. They took off and ran 1 lap in 2 minutes, and I told them to stop. A lap in 2 minutes was plenty, so I briefed them on another test:

WITH BODY ARMOR, 3 ROUNDS OF:

RUN I LAP WITH THE WORM

10 BURPEES OVER THE HAY BALE IN PAIRS

I also told them to be prepared for the challenge to change mid-event—I might add reps or rounds. The first run took 1:58, and the first set of 10 burpees took 1:50. They finished the entire round in 3:50, including transition time.

The rest of the rounds were finished at a similar pace. The last 2 runs were around 2:30, and the burpees took around 1:45-2:00 each round.

After finishing Round 3, they looked pretty exhausted. I told them to do one more round. That was at the 12:45 mark. As they picked up the Worm and started to run, Jacob Wilson from Rogue yelled, *"Just one more! Here you go!"* After they were gone, I told him that actually might not be true. We all laughed.

Once they got back and finished the round, I told them to do a fifth, which would be the final round. They finished the test in 22:20.

I don't know where I am with this one. I have mixed feelings on it, largely because of their response. One of the team members said it wasn't too bad. Others said it hurt. In a race environment, though, you go fast and they always hurt. I might increase the reps a little on the burpees. I need to process this one a little more.

*Sunday, June 25, 2:10 p.m.*

I've been at Yarrow for a few hours today. I leave tomorrow on the big Madison trip, so I need to get a bunch of stuff done. I did some Team planning—not much—and then dove into the Individual schedule. I updated the board where I have all the workouts and movements laid out. I noticed a lot of loaded components—13—and not as many gymnastics components—seven. I also noticed I have a ton of couplets and triplets—five couplets and three triplets. That's not necessarily a bad thing. Couplets and triplets are at the heart of CrossFit, and they're essentially the foundation of effective programming. I currently have no chipper. Well, the Banger is technically a couplet chipper, but I mean I don't have a traditional chipper.

I see all this as an opportunity to make positive changes. The row workout with the GHD and the push presses would be a good place for a chipper. As I started playing it out, I came up with a gymnastics-heavy chipper. This is what I sketched out: 80 pull-ups, 70 GHD sit-ups, 60 toes-to-bars, 50 pistols, 30 push presses. I could still add the row in there, too. So it would essentially be a G-G-G-G-M-W event.

*(In CrossFit, G represents a gymnastics movement, basically a body-weight movement. M is monostructural, including things like rowing, running, swimming, etc.—classic "cardio." W is weightlifting, which encompasses all movements that include loading with an object.)*

I like that: G *(pull-ups)*, G *(GHD)*, G *(toes-to-bars)*, G *(pistols)*, M *(rowing)*, W *(push presses with 100-lb. dumbbells).*

*Monday, June 26, 3:04 p.m.*

I'm currently on a Southwest flight to Milwaukee. There is no direct flight to Madison from San Diego. I have to fly to Chicago, Denver or Utah and then take a second flight to Madison.

It's a one-hour drive to the San Diego airport and a two-hour flight to the first location. Usually the layover is an hour, and then it's two hours to Madison. But Southwest does have a direct flight to Milwaukee, so I decided to give that a try. I'll fly into Milwaukee, meet with Milwaukee-based affiliates that evening, and then go to the Harley-Davidson Museum Tuesday morning before heading to Madison.

*Wednesday, June 28, 5:21 p.m.*

I had a really busy couple of days in Wisconsin.

The affiliate gathering on Tuesday evening went well. I met a lot of people and hosted a small Q&A session, mostly about the Games. I think they enjoyed it, and I had fun. The Harley-Davidson tour was great. That museum is really nice and very large, full of unique motorcycles and interactive displays. They did a great job putting that museum together.

Once I got to Madison on Tuesday, we went over the venue. I had Chase Ingraham waiting to test the Run-Swim-Run. Whenever I have swim events, I try to get Chase involved in the testing. Chase swam in college, and he also participated in triathlons before getting into CrossFit. And he's a great CrossFit athlete, so it makes sense for him to test the water events. He also has a really good attitude and is a fun guy to be around.

I briefed him on the event and then discussed timing. I thought the 500-meter swim could be done in 5-6 minutes, but he said not in open lake water. He predicted about 8-9 minutes. He said a good rule of thumb is 1:30 for 100 meters in water like this for good swimmers.

Justin and I got on bikes—the bikes we used at the triathlon we did at the Games years ago—and we led Chase on the course.

**RUN 1.5 MILES**

**SWIM 500 METERS**

**RUN 1.5 MILES**

The first .8 miles or so is all on the campus of the venue, and the next .5 miles or so is on a trail system. Chase was running relatively fast and hit the end of the run at 10:10. His transition to the water took him about 15 seconds. As he entered the slip, he actually took a nice fall onto the ground. He picked himself up and continued into the water. And off he went.

His pace in the water seemed good. It's always hard to tell how fast someone is swimming when he or she is solo and you don't really have reference markers for distance. He made it to the first-turn buoy at 12:30. There, he made a right turn into a long, straight length. He made it to the final buoy at the 15:45 mark and turned to return to land. On the final leg, there were a couple of moments when he kind of pulled up and looked around. It looked like he was briefly resting, but in reality he was just getting his bearing straight. Chase exited the water at 19:52, making his total swim time for the 500 9:26—right around the time he predicted. His transition on the way out was a little slower—34 seconds. On the run back, he pushed hard and was moving as fast as he could considering what he had done already. He ended up crossing the finish line at 31:03, meaning about 10:31 for his second 1.5 miles. That was slightly slower than his 10:10 on the way out, but it was still a great time coming back.

We let him recover for a bit, then talked about the event and how he felt. He said it was a great test, and the combo was a nice touch. He felt light-headed getting out of the water to start his second run. We agreed some people would really struggle.

Later in the evening, I texted with him to ask how many people he thinks will beat his time. He said about 50 percent of the men. I also wondered how many will go sub 30, and he said about 10 or so. Sub 30 will be moving. Call it 10 minutes for each mile and a half and then a sub-10 swim.

After having Chase test, I'm very excited about the event. I think it will provide a great opening test for the athletes and some spectacular races. It will be really interesting to have the Age Group athletes and the teams go through, too. On the low end we'll see high 20s for the time. On the high end, we might see 40s to 50s. Either way, it will be entertaining.

That evening we went to CrossFit Madtown, where we hosted an affiliate dinner and workout. The workout was first, and it was for all the affiliate owners from the Madison area—the same group we regularly get together with. Chase and I programmed the workout. I was originally leaning in the direction of something that had a barbell, but with around 50 or more people, it made sense to avoid the barbell. The workout we settled on was run 400 meters, 100 paired push-ups in groups of four (two people do synchronized push-ups and the other two rest, working back and forth in pairs to 100 reps), run 400 meters, 100 air squats in the same fashion, run 400 meters, 100 burpees, and a final 400-meter run.

Chase's team was strong. They had Johnny Mac and a couple of other good guys, and they finished in 14 minutes. My team did well. We finished around 17 minutes, and I think we were fifth out of about 11 or 12 teams.

This morning we had our big meeting to announce the events to the team and the people most critical to running the competition that is the CrossFit Games. It started at 9, and the first thing I made clear was the fact that 90 percent of the Individual workouts are done, but there is a 100 percent certainty that 50 percent of them will change. For the teams, 50 percent are done, with a 100 percent certainty that 90 percent of them will change.

With that out of the way, we looked at the big-picture schedule, then dug into the Individual competition. That took an hour. After that, we dug into the Team competition. Then we looked at the Team and Individual schedules in detail to see how they worked together. After that, we took a look at the Age Group events and how they all play together. I had Pat brief those as we looked at each event.

Throughout, we brought up concerns and issues for gear and events. Bill and Caity Henniger from Rogue were there, so we had a lot to bounce off them.

After we finished all those tasks, we walked around the campus and took a look at the various areas. The Coliseum is coming together great. When I walked in, I commented on how something looked different. It turns out they had painted the piss-yellow paint white, and that really freshened it up. It was a nice touch. We then walked out to the north lot, where our outdoor competition will be set up, and we saw the true size of the area. It will be large—not as large as the Soccer Stadium in Carson but large enough. The visual was very nice, with all areas having cones to represent where the bleachers would be, where the floor would be, etc.

So far, it's been a great trip. Tonight we have a dinner with our crew, and then tomorrow I have a half day of media obligations before I leave at 12. I'm not really looking forward to that, but it's something I need to do to promote the sport and help it grow.

*Thursday, June 29, 4:17 p.m.*
I'm currently flying home from Milwaukee on a direct flight to San Diego. Today was a long morning of interviews with our media and local Madison media. It started off with a 7-a.m. interview with Rory McKernan and our team about the Games. That one will be for some of the CBS pieces and promos for our outlets. I enjoyed it—it was an easy, fun chat.

Next, I met with our POCs from the Madison city commission and Scott Panchik. Scott was in town to help us with some of the local PR and promos we were supposed to do. Scott is someone I've really enjoyed hanging out with over the years. I would say we're friends, but I wouldn't say we're as close as I am with Rich Froning, Dan Bailey or Josh Bridges.

We drove over to HotelRED and walked into the lobby. I did an interview over the phone with a local radio station first. This one was quick and pretty easy, nothing challenging or stimulating. After that, I figured we were meeting with a couple of people at the RED for our next media requirement. Then I saw a large group of people, probably 50-60, and I asked why they were here. Our host replied that they were here for a large Q&A session about the Games. I didn't quite realize that. Jeb Simmons was also there. He's the local Madison athlete who qualified for the Games in the 40-44 Division.

The session was fun. We sat in front of the group of about 60 and a moderator asked us a variety of questions. Then audience members were allowed to ask us questions. At one point, the moderator asked how we would each "*pitch*" CrossFit to the group. When it came to me, I said I am not a pitch man, and it's not my job to try to sell CrossFit to anybody.

After that, we drove to one of the three local TV stations and did an individual interview with a gentleman who had done his homework and had legitimate questions. I enjoyed this interaction. The next stops were at the other local TV stations, and I did not enjoy those at all. One was a sit-down interview with a local TV anchor and Scott. It was very conservative and tame. She didn't know anything about us really, and it felt like a waste of my time. The second interview was even worse. It was a quick chat with a guy who vaguely looked like he belonged on "*Anchorman*." He had not done his homework, either. I was officially over it. Luckily, that was our last media obligation. Unlike some who really thrive in that environment or seek out that attention, I really don't. I will do it for the team and to support our sport, but it's not my thing.

When we were in the car driving around to the different venues and interviews, Scott and I had a talk about something I've been chatting about with others over the last few days: the elusive combination of the 500-lb. back squat and sub-5-minute mile. We talked about who we thought could do it. Scott said his back squat is over 500 but his mile is not close to sub 5. We guessed at Rich's back squat and agreed it was around 475. I texted Rich and he confirmed it—something he hasn't tested in over a year, he said. Apparently Garret Fisher is close to the goal. He is a large guy, so the 500+ back squat does not surprise me. Garret is actually one of the faster runners in the field of top CrossFit athletes, so a sub-5 mile is not so much of a surprise to me. I told Scott the standard should be a 500-lb. back squat, a sub-5 mile and something like 50 pull-ups unbroken. The 50 pull-ups would really establish that it's a CrossFit athlete who sets this record. I think there could be some strong types—maybe decathletes—who could maybe do the 500/sub 5. Either way, it's very interesting. Maybe we'll have the opportunity to test it sometime in the near future.

I'm looking forward to getting back home and essentially finishing the programming. I'll spend tomorrow and this weekend on some in-depth testing with the new group of athletes coming in: Alex Parker, Kelley Jackson and Paul Tremblay. I'm really interested in having the women test some of the events.

*8:47 p.m.*

I called an audible today. I landed in San Diego at 4:40. While I was driving home, I called Justin and was debriefing the events of the past few days. Before I got off the phone, I told him I was excited to test with Paul, Alex and Kelley tomorrow. He mentioned he thought they should all be there tonight. So I thought, *"Great. Let's test something tonight so I can really maximize my time with them."* I texted Stephane and told him to ask them if they could test at 7:30. They of course agreed. I went home, said hello to the family, had dinner with them, spent a little time unpacking and then drove to Yarrow to meet them.

Stephane and I discussed what we should have them test, and I decided on Long Amanda—13-11-9-7-5. Just Alex and Kelley. Not Paul. From Julian's test, I think I have enough data to know what I need to do for the men. But I wanted to see what the times would be for women. I asked both ladies about their muscle-ups. Alex said they're a weakness and Kelley said they're a strength. That actually works well for testing purposes. They both warmed up and looked great on the 95-lb. snatches. That obviously won't be an issue for them or the women at the Games.

I had them both do this at the same time:

13-11-9-7-5 REPS OF:

RING MUSCLE-UPS

SQUAT SNATCHES (95 LB.)

Kelley was stronger on the rings than Alex. That was obvious on the first set. Kelley only broke it up into 3 sets and finished 13 muscle-ups in

1:10. Alex broke it up a few more times and finished in 1:55. Kelley finished her first round in 2:19, and Alex finished in 3:09.

The round of 11 muscle-ups started to slow them both down. Kelley finished that set at 3:54, almost 3 minutes faster than Alex, who finished at 6:54. Kelley finished her set of 11 snatches at 5:32, and Alex finished hers at 8:07.

On Round 3, which is essentially the start of the Amanda part of the test, Kelley finished the muscle-ups at 7:42. Alex was done at 10:34. Kelley finished the set of 9 squat snatches at 9:17 to Alex's 11:46. Both ladies moved the bar well and usually in big sets. I'm not sure, but I think Alex did larger sets than Kelley, probably just to try to close the gap a little.

Kelley attacked the final 2 rounds and finished the set of 7 muscle-ups at 11:13. She was done with 7 squat snatches at 12:36. She then finished 5 muscle-ups at 13:46, and she completed the test at 14:47. She would have been much faster, but there was some miscommunication between us, and she was under the impression she had to do a set of 3 muscle-ups and 3 squat snatches. I think she would have been low 14s if she had realized the 5s were her last round.

Alex, on the other hand, started to really struggle with the muscle-ups. She finished the set of 7 at 14:19, then ripped the set of 7 snatches to end the round near the 15-minute mark. I just told her to stop at that point.

My original intent was to have a time cap of 12 minutes for both men and women. Having seen these ladies do it, I think 12 minutes is too aggressive for the women. It's likely still appropriate for the men, but I should probably use a 15-minute cap for the women.

I'm really glad we called this audible and tested tonight. It quickly forced me back into the testing and planning routine I had to leave when I went to Madison. We have a great few days ahead of us. I don't know Alex and Kelley that well, but it seems like they'll be fun to hang with and get to know. I know Paul well because he's on our Level 1 Seminar Staff team and has worked with me a lot in the past on our Demo Team. He was also an Individual Games competitor in 2014. I like his attitude and his style. We get along well.

*9:10 p.m.*

One last important entry for tonight. During all my media obligations today in Madison, I saw a concept for a great Games event in 2018. I can't talk about it here because this book will be out before those Games. But it's something that will stick and go through revisions in my mind 100 times before the 2018 competition. I'll figure out if we can do it and how it should look.

*Friday, June 30, 4:46 p.m.*

This morning I met up with the Demo Team at 9 a.m. First, I had them test a new version of the Friday chipper. I had both ladies work up to the 70-lb. dumbbell in warm-up. At first they both struggled with it, especially Kelley. But then she gained some confidence and was able to cycle it well. I decided to have Kelley do it instead of Alex because Kelley is the smaller of the two. I wanted to see how the 70 would treat her. Paul had no issue cycling the 100, but I never questioned that he would. I was going to have them both go at the same time. It's three gymnastics movements, a mono-structural movement that favors bigger athletes, and a heavy weightlifting movement, so it would be good to see both athletes do it.

80 PULL-UPS

70 GHD SIT-UPS

60 PISTOLS

40 CALORIES ON THE CONCEPT2

20 PUSH PRESSES (100/70 LB.)

They both ripped out large sets of pull-ups to start. Kelley did a set of 50, and Paul did a set of 45. Both took 45 seconds. Kelley then did 20 and 10 to finish at 1:31. Paul did a set that took him to 66, then a third set that took him to 80. He finished a few seconds before Kelley.

Before we started, Paul had said he would be slow on the GHD. I would find out later that he had injured his adductor before Regionals and hasn't really done much for GHD work since. It showed here. He finished 70 at 5:32, with Kelley a minute ahead at 4:32. Kelley had finished roughly 30 pistols before Paul got off the GHD.

When Paul first started the pistols, he struggled a bit. He was out of rhythm and didn't have his balance. Kelley had gone right into them with no issues and was knocking out big sets with short breaks. She finished the set of 70 pistols at 6:50. Paul finished at 8:38, almost 2 minutes behind her.

This is when things changed and it got interesting. Even though Kelley started about 2 minutes ahead of Paul on the rower, she finished at 9:43 to his 10:36. Because of the significant size difference between the two, he made up a bunch of time on her. Of course I understand this was not a race between him and her. But their times allow me to get a sense of how smaller athletes and bigger athletes would perform. The larger competitors might be able to make big moves on this section, as Paul was doing.

Kelley got to the shoulders-to-overheads at 10:08. It took her until 10:25 to get 5 on her right arm, and then she moved forward and switched to her left. The next 5 took her from 10:44 to 11:39, and she missed a couple. At 10:52, Paul made it to his dumbbell, picked it up and did a set of 10. He put it down at 11:17, then picked it back up and finished another set of 10 for a total time of 11:58. Kelley finished her third set exactly as Paul finished the test, and it her took roughly a minute to do her final reps. She finished at 12:54.

At one point, Paul had been almost 2 minutes behind. But because of the row and his ability to manhandle the 100, he beat Kelley by almost a minute.

I like how this version played out. I'm going to leave it for now. I don't think I'll change much at this point, but I will analyze it later with the other events when I look at the big picture to see if anything needs to be altered.

After we finished that, I asked Alex to warm up for the bar-muscle-up/clean event. We discussed weights. Alex said her 1RM is around 230, so I didn't expect her to get too far into the 200 bars. We came up with this:

8 ROUNDS OF:

4 BAR MUSCLE-UPS

2 CLEANS (145, 160, 175, 190, 205, 215, 225, 235 LB.)

She got through the first 4 bars in 3:20, with unbroken muscle-ups. In the fifth round, she broke the muscle-ups into 2 sets of 2. Both lifts at 190 looked really difficult. She got under them but was very slow coming out of the hole. On 205, she was able to get under but could not stand. She made 2 attempts, and after the second I called her off.

I think the weight is appropriate for the women. Alex and Kelley are both on the smaller side. I'm not worried about whether the larger girls can handle that weight.

Julian showed up while Alex was doing that event, so we played some great games of knockout a few minutes after Alex finished. The girls actually did great. Each won a few rounds. I think I heard them say Kelley actually played basketball in college. Or maybe it was high school.

I decided to have Julian test a version of Sunday's event with 2-minute intervals. A week ago, we tested a version with the Concept2 rower and pistols. We scratched the pistols and decided to pull the rower because of the time it takes to get in and out of it.

4 2-MINUTE ROUNDS OF:

2 LEGLESS ROPE CLIMBS

15 CALORIES ON THE SKIERG

AMRAP OHS (135 LB.) IN THE REMAINING TIME TO 75 TOTAL

REST 1 MINUTE BETWEEN ROUNDS

On the first round, Julian finished the legless rope climbs in 22 seconds, he finished 15 calories at 1:09, and he did 20 OHS in the remaining time.

On the second round, he did the rope climbs in 27 seconds and completed the 15 calories at 1:27. He got 13 squats in the remaining time for a total of 33 in 2 rounds. I decided 15 would be too many, but I didn't change it on him during this test. I also decided it should be standard rope climbs with legs. I want to keep those elements fast so it's more about the squats at the end. On the second round, he only had 30 seconds of time to work on squats.

Julian did the third round with his legs and finished in 25 seconds. He finished the calories around 1:25, and he knocked out 12 OHS in the remaining time for a total of 45.

On the final round he completed the climbs and the 15 cals at 1:42. He was able to get an additional 6 OHS for a total of 51.

The 15 calories took too long. I would prefer if athletes had time to do some real work on the bar, even in the final round. The other thing to remember is that the athletes will have to run across the floor to do the work at the Games. That's another reason to ensure the stuff in the beginning is consistently fast.

We talked for a minute, and I asked Paul if he wanted to give it a go. He said for sure. I decided he could use his legs on the climb, but this was a short rope like the one we used at Regionals, so you can't use your legs right away. It's a "*hybrid*" rope climb. I wanted him to do 10 calories instead of 15, and I decided to up the weight a tad. We moved it to 155.

**4 2-MINUTE ROUNDS OF:**

**2 ROPE CLIMBS**

**10 CALORIES ON THE SKIERG**

**AMRAP OHS (155 LB.) IN THE REMAINING TIME TO 75 TOTAL**

**REST 1 MINUTE BETWEEN ROUNDS**

On the first round, he finished the first two components at 52 seconds, whereas Julian had finished them at 1:09. With the remaining time, Paul was able to get 21 squats. He actually stopped at 20 and dropped the bar, then picked it back up and got another, but he stopped at 1:52. I don't know what he was doing there.

On the second round, he finished the first two parts in 1:01. Julian had finished those in 1:27. I liked our new changes. Paul was able to get 18 reps in the remaining time for a total of 39.

On the third round, he finished the first two parts in 1:10 to Julian's 1:28 or so. With the remaining time, Paul squeezed in 12 reps to reach 51.

On the fourth round, he finished the first two parts in 1:15 to Julian's 1:42. This solidified it: The changes were just what I wanted. Paul got an additional 13 reps in the final round for 64 total. Of note, he finished 60 at 1:48 in the last round. That's good to know as I consider the final total rep count for this test.

After that, we played some more knockout before I took the crew to lunch. Kelley and Alex are cool people, and I enjoy hanging out with them.

I learned that Alex just finished law school. She also trains with Michael FitzGerald. He's been around CrossFit for a long time. We go way back to the early years of the Games.

Kelley and her husband run an affiliate, CrossFit Gambit. She worked at Reebok for two years before leaving that job to open the affiliate.

After lunch, I told them to take a break before we meet up again at 4:30.

*7:19 p.m.*

This afternoon, the first thing we did was change out the rope. We took down the short Regional rope that forces you to do a few legless pulls before you have enough rope to use your legs. That was an ordeal. We had to stack a tall ladder on some foam boxes, and I climbed up. It was very sketchy. But we got the 20-foot rope in place.

I told Kelley to warm up for the same event that I had Julian and Paul do. We decided on 8 calories for her and 105 lb. for the weight. She would also have the full-length rope so she could use her legs the entire time.

**4 2-MINUTE ROUNDS OF:**

**2 ROPE CLIMBS**

**8 CALORIES ON THE SKIERG**

**AMRAP OHS (105 LB.) IN THE REMAINING TIME TO 75 TOTAL**

**REST 1 MINUTE BETWEEN ROUNDS**

Kelley finished the first pair of movements at 1:05 and completed 21 unbroken squats in the remaining time. She has great positioning and moves well. On the second round, she finished the first two movements in 1:09, then went on to hit 19 squats (*40 total*).

On the third round, Kelley finished the first two sections in 1:15, then got 16 squats (*56 total*).

On the final round she finished the first two pieces at 1:27, then performed 11 squats for a total of 67. If we used 60 as the total, she would have finished right around 1:47.

I'm thinking of maybe even dropping the calories on the female version to 7 just to speed it up. I might have Alex test it tomorrow with 7 instead. I need some time to process before having her test it.

Speaking of Alex, I decided to have her test something else. Earlier in the day, she mentioned she's a strong runner, so I decided to have her test the hay-bale event. Julian did it in 18:30. I didn't think her time would be faster but wanted to see what a fast female competitor could do.

5 ROUNDS OF:

RUN 500 METERS

9 CLEANS (70-LB. D-BALL) OVER THE HAY BALES PLUS BURPEES OVER THE BALES

Alex took off at a very fast pace and finished the run in 1:55. She looked slow and reserved on the cleans and ended up finishing the first round at 3:24. I thought she would eventually slow up and fail to beat Julian's time.

She finished her second round at 6:47 for a round time of 3:23—almost the same as her first.

Her third round was complete at 10:22 with a round time of 3:35. Her cleans and burpees were starting to improve, and she was really moving in that section.

Her fourth round was complete at 14:06 with a round time of 3:44—her slowest yet. But she was now on pace to beat Julian's time of 18:30.

Alex ended up finishing the fifth round at 17:47—3:41 for the round. I was really impressed. She's a great runner. Her running speed makes me consider bumping the test up a little. I considered doing that after Julian's test, but not just with a longer run—perhaps with more in the clean/burpee section. Maybe I'll make it 11 reps instead of 9. I might have Paul test this one in the next few days.

Overall, it was a great testing day. We got a lot of work done, and I have some good data to play with. I told them to meet up tomorrow at 9 a.m. for another full day of testing. Each did two events today. Tomorrow I hope to have each do three.

## JULY 2017

*Saturday, July 1, 2:12 p.m.*

We met at 9 a.m. this morning. I didn't realize it was Canada Day, and I didn't really know what Canada Day is. Kelley was poking fun at our Canadians, Alex and Paul, and I learned that July 1 is their equivalent to the Fourth of July. I also learned that 2017 marks the 150th anniversary of Canada, so it was a big day for them. But instead of being home celebrating, they were with me in California testing out potential CrossFit Games events.

The first thing I had them test was the odd-object/handstand-walk event. We had to pull out a lot of equipment and weights, and we measured a 90-foot length outside my building. Most days it's sunny and very hot, but it was an overcast morning with a tinge of humidity—a perfect time to test.

We started with Paul. We played around and ended up with a total yoke weight of 420 lb. At the Games two years ago, the yoke weighed 380. Next, we loaded the farmers-carry handles we had with one blue plate *(45 lb.)* and one green *(25 lb.)* on each end. We put four reds *(55 lb. each)* on a sled.

After we were all loaded up, I explained the event, and they were very excited. They had to move every object 90 feet across the floor, using a handstand walk to return to get the next object. Then they had to return everything back to its original place. It ends up being six trips across with an object and four walks of 90 feet. At Regionals, we had athletes do four walks of 60 feet, so I like the increased distance here.

### MOVE YOKE, FARMERS-CARRY HANDLES AND SLED ACROSS FLOOR

### *HANDSTAND WALK WHEN MOVING BACK

On go, Paul pulled the sled across the floor in 16 seconds. He broke his handstand walk back across the floor once. At 1:02, he had essentially completed one full round. Next, he chose the farmers carry. It took him around 29 seconds to get across. His second handstand walk was slower than the first: It took him a full minute to do it in 3 sets.

The third object presents an opportunity: Once you get the object across, you don't have to follow with a handstand walk. You just take one of the objects back. Paul chose to take the yoke last so he could walk it across, stop, turn around and walk it right back. The whole process took him 36 seconds, but it affected him significantly on the next handstand walk. His third walk took him 1:30 in 4 sets. (*Afterward, he mentioned it was a bad idea to go from yoke to handstand walk because of how much it taxed his core and midline stability.*)

Next, he took the handles back in about 14 seconds. On his fourth and final handstand walk, he again used 4 sets, and it took him 1:24. Finally, he pulled the sled back in about 20 seconds for a total time of 7:55, including rest and transition time.

I was surprised his handstand walks took so much time. I told the ladies they would do it next, and I figured they would be much faster.

Alex went first. She got under a 300-lb. yoke to start—we had used the same weight at the Games in 2015. The yoke took her 28 seconds. Her first handstand walk was broken into 3 sets and complete at 1:35.

Next, she carried the handles. She broke the following handstand walk into 4 sets, and the round was finished at 3:38.

She decided to pull the sled, then move the handles back, and she crossed the line at 4:37. Things started to get really tough here. She struggled to complete the handstand walk: It took 5 sets and almost 3 minutes. She moved the sled, then broke her final handstand walk into 6 sets that took a little over 2 minutes. She carried her yoke across the line at the 10-minute mark.

I was surprised. I had expected her to do much better than Paul, but she struggled with the handstand walks.

Next up was Kelley, and I used the same loads. I was hoping—and kinda expecting—that Kelley would crush Paul's time, but I was proved wrong.

Kelley chose the sled first and ran it across the floor. She broke her first walk into 3 sets, and the first pair of movements took 1:03.

She carried the handles next and broke the handstand walk into 4 sets, but it still only took about a minute. She took the yoke across, then pulled the sled back to its original position. The third handstand walk cost her a lot of time. It took almost 2 minutes, whereas her first ones were a minute or less each. She broke the third walk up 5 times, then carried the handles back. Her final walk was actually kind of fast compared to her third. It took about 1:20 even though she broke it up 9 times. I was really surprised by that. The breaks were super quick, though. She would kick up, come down and kick right back up. Once she finished that set, she carried the yoke across the finish line for a total time of 7:59—4 seconds slower than Paul. To my surprise, Paul's time stood.

The odd objects taxed the handstand walk much more than I thought they would. But this still seems like an appropriate event and test. I think it will be very exciting and very challenging. There isn't much use testing it more here. I have some good baseline info, but we need to test it in Madison on the actual floor with the actual equipment.

The sled will likely be a different Rogue model, and it will move differently on the artificial turf we're laying in Madison. The handles will be different, too. They're making a version of Slaters Hardware handles for us.

I originally had this as a quick event with a 6-minute cap, but I need to increase that. I could only use two objects and make it 2 walks across, but I like using 3, so we'll continue with that plan.

After a short break, I decided to have them test the final event. I had Paul go first and test this:

12-10-8 REPS OF:

HANDSTAND PUSH-UPS ON PARALLETTES

KETTLEBELL DEADLIFTS (200 LB.)

THEN:

LUNGE 2 53-LB. KETTLEBELLS 80 FEET

Paul did all sets of handstand push-ups unbroken, and he broke every round of deadlifts into 2 sets. His total time for that first couplet was 3:30. He then picked up the 2 lighter kettlebells and literally screamed as he went 15 feet and came crashing to the ground. He completed 80 feet in 4 sets for a total time of 7:18. After he finished the test, he fell to the ground and writhed in pain. He said this was the hardest one he has tested yet.

I decided to have Kelley test it with 150-lb. kettlebells. She did 12 HSPU unbroken, then used sets of 8 and 4 deadlifts to finish the first round in 1:15.

On her second set of HSPU, she started to struggle, and I realized 12-10-8 reps might slow it down too much. I told her just to do 9, and I was going to change the scheme to 12-9-6. She did 9 in about a minute—triple the time it had taken her to do the set of 12. She spent a minute on 3 sets of deadlifts.

She used sets of 4 and 2 to complete the last HSPU, and she did the deadlifts in 2 sets—but with a lot of rest. Her total time at this point was 5:03.

Kelley had better luck with the lunges than Paul did. With 35 lb. in each hand, she completed one length, put them down, turned around and came back to finish at 7:18.

She, too, went to the floor and later talked about how hard it was. I think this will be appropriate as a final, but I still need to make some changes.

I had Alex do it next but subbed in the 124-lb. kettlebells we used two years ago at the Games. I was most interested in speeding up the first couplet, and Alex finished that part in 4:50, about 2 seconds faster than Kelley. (*Alex later said the handstand push-ups were much harder because they did 360 feet of handstand walking an hour prior. That makes total sense.*) She finished the entire test in 6:28.

After watching the tests, I realized a couple of things need to happen: I need to test with the actual parallettes we'll use at the Games, and I need to play with the reps to see if I can make it faster. When we were talking about options, I presented a 10-9-8 version. It's the same rep total, but the scheme might entice you to do the first set of kettlebell deadlifts unbroken. I'll have Julian test that version this week. Or maybe one of these guys tomorrow. Not sure yet.

Overall, it was another great morning of testing. I'm getting ready to head back there within the hour to have them test some more stuff. This will be all for the day, I think. They have each done two good events so far.

*8:38 p.m.*

I just had dinner with the crew. I took them to West Steak and Seafood in Carlsbad. My wife trains the head chef from time to time. The ambiance is nice, and it was a great dinner.

This afternoon, we met at 3:30 for the second testing sessions. I won't soon forget this afternoon. I saw some performances that left me speechless.

First, we loaded up 6 bars so Paul could test the muscle-up/clean event. (We only loaded up 6 bars and would add change plates to the last one to get to the final loads.) I asked him what his 1RM clean was, and he said 390.

"OK, so he should be able to finish this one," I figured.

Julian's 1RM is 365. He got 1 at 350 and didn't finish in the 10-minute cap, but his performance was strong.

After we had all the bars set up, Paul and I spoke about the time and the plan. I said I expect the top guys to be in the range of 6-7 minutes. I didn't mention this to him, but I figured he would finish it in 8-9.

8 ROUNDS OF:

4 BAR MUSCLE-UPS

2 CLEANS (225, 245, 265, 285, 305, 320, 335, 350 LB.)

Paul started out quick but not fast. He did all sets of bar muscle-ups unbroken. The bar muscle-ups are not meant to be incredibly challenging. They are meant to be more of an annoyance. Really, this event is a test of strength. Paul did the first round in 25 seconds.

He completed the second round at 1:05. Again, he was not rushed. He was deliberate.

His third round was done at 1:41.

He finished Round 4 at 2:24. He had used power cleans for all the bars up to this point.

He finished the round with 305 lb. at 3:08 and the 320-lb. round at 4:02—all with power cleans. I was baffled by how smooth he was moving and his impressive time. There was no sense of urgency, yet he was killing it.

On his seventh round, he power-cleaned the first one at 335 but had to drop lower than before. On the second rep, he used a squat clean. He finished that round at 4:57.

He used a pair of squat cleans to finish the test in 5:57.

I was blown away. I didn't expect him to be so fast. I imagine his score today will be one of the faster times at the Games. I'm excited about this event. I'm happy with the changes I made and where it's ending up.

In this year's testing so far, Paul's effort was the most impressive feat—but something more impressive was about to go down.

I had Alex do the interval event next. The big change: I dropped the SkiErg to 7 calories for the women, and I made a big change to the timing of the rounds. I had this idea earlier on and wanted to experiment with it. Basically, everything is the same, but on the final round, you get 3 minutes instead of 2. You can still build up a lead in the first rounds and have an advantage going in, but this format makes the last round the true deciding factor. In the original version, you just didn't have that much time to get work done. In this version, I could increase the total reps. I don't remember why or how I came up with this idea. It just popped into my head. I think this longer final round will play well.

I told Alex about the new plan, and she understood.

### 3 2-MINUTE ROUNDS AND 1 3-MINUTE ROUND OF:

### 2 ROPE CLIMBS

### 7 CALORIES ON THE SKIERG

### AS MANY OHS (105 LB.) AS POSSIBLE IN REMAINING TIME (TOTAL REPS UNKNOWN)

Alex ripped up the rope, finishing both climbs in 28 seconds. She finished with the SkiErg at 1:08. In the remaining time, she was able to do 20 unbroken squats. Her squat looked great. Often, athletes without ideal positioning will fight with this movement, especially at high reps, but she has good form, which would pay off in the later rounds.

On Round 2, after a minute of rest, she finished the first two parts of the test in 1:03, about 5 seconds faster than the previous round. In her remaining time, she got 17 squats for a total of 37. Her pace slowed a little on the OHS but not as much as I expected. She only did 3 fewer.

After her 1-minute rest, she attacked the third round. She finished the 2 rope climbs in 34 seconds and then left the SkiErg at 1:08. In her remaining time, she squeaked in 15 overhead squats—again unbroken—to bring her total to 52.

The next round featured the big change to a 3-minute cap. Alex finished the rope climbs in 36 seconds, then finished the calories at 1:14. It was her slowest split, which was to be expected in the final round. She picked up the bar and did 8 squats for a total of 60 at the 1:40 mark. I told her to go to 70. She put her bar down, rested for a second and started again. She did a set of 10 and hit the 70-rep total at 2:20. She dropped the bar again, and after a few seconds of rest she asked if I wanted her to continue. I said no. I had seen enough. I probably should have had her go on. My mistake for stopping her. In the end, I still saw enough to know how I need to test it again.

Finally, I asked Kelley if she was good at thrusters and double-unders. She shrugged and said, "Yeah, pretty good." I asked her how she did in 17.5, and she said, "OK. I think it was top 20 in the world."

Top 20 in the world—just OK. That's amazing.

She was actually ninth in the world on that event. When I said she was going to do 17.5 with 95 lb., her eyes lit up. I got excited because she was excited, and the feeling spread. The energy in our small testing group was incredible. It was go time.

She warmed up and got ready for the test, and we were all wondering how fast she would be. I told them Julian had done it in about 11 minutes.

10 ROUNDS OF:

9 THRUSTERS AT 95 LB.

35 DOUBLE-UNDERS

Kelley started at a great pace and did the first round in 42 seconds. Her pace and movement were consistent.

She finished the second round at 1:28.

Hardly slowing up, she finished the first 5 rounds at 3:58. And at this point, I realized she had the potential to go sub 10. That was unbelievable to me. She stayed consistent and just kept chipping away, taking very few breaks.

It wasn't until the sixth round or so that she started collecting herself before proceeding. She would take an extra breath or so before picking up the rope or doing thrusters.

She finished the eighth round at 7:22 and the ninth at 8:35. At this point, I was confident she would be under 10. She hadn't broken anything in 9 rounds. Not a single set of thrusters or double-unders.

In her 10th round, she put the bar down at 9:05, 5 reps into the thrusters. I was so surprised. *"Damn, now she won't get sub 10,"* I thought. She quickly picked the bar up and did the remaining reps, finishing the thrusters at 9:31. She had 29 seconds to get to her rope and finish 35 double-unders. I didn't think it would happen, but she did that final set of 35 at a pace I hadn't seen her use before. She finished all 35 and fell to the floor with 9:54 on the clock!

We were all blown away. Her time puts her in the 95th percentile in the world of all men who did 17.5 as Rx'd in the Open. Kelley was ninth on 17.5 in the Open, and some of the girls who beat her will be at the Games: Camille Leblanc-Bazinet, Brooke Wells, Sara Sigmundsdottir and Kristin Holte. That's great. It sets up some fireworks at the Games. Some of the girls will for sure go sub 10 unless they are too beat up by that point—but I don't think they will be.

Of all the testing performances to this stage, this was one of the most exciting and impressive I've seen. This event will be great at the Games. I can't wait for it.

Tomorrow is our last day of testing before the three of them leave. I'll try to get a few more events in and then cut them away for the rest of the day.

*Sunday, July 2, 4:15 p.m.*
We were supposed to meet at 9 a.m. this morning, but I slept in and then had to squeeze in the CrossFit.com WOD: 5 rounds of swim 200 meters and rest 2 minutes. I was still sore from Barbara two days ago. The first swim went fine. I pushed hard, but my lats and arms were on fire for the rest of the swimming. The intervals got really hard, and I got slow. I'm still feeling it hours later.

We eventually met at 9:30 a.m. Once I showed up, we shot the shit a little and then got into testing.

First, I wanted to have Kelley test the run/clean/burpee event. I needed someone small to test it to see how the height of the hay bales would affect the event. I also increased the reps by 2. Julian and Alex had done 9 each round.

5 ROUNDS OF:

RUN 500 M

II CLEANS (70 LB.) OVER THE HAY BALES PLUS BURPEES OVER THE BALES

Kelley finished the first round in 3:31, whereas Alex had finished in 3:24.

Kelley's runs were slower than Alex's, but her cleans and burpees over the hay were faster. The 2 extra reps leveled out that section.

By the end of Round 4, the comparison looked like this: 15:59 for Kelley and 14:06 for Alex.

Alex had completed the event by the time Kelley got in from her fifth run. Kelley tried to go sub 20 but slipped with a clean and almost dropped the bag. Her total time was 20:01. Alex's time from two days ago—with 10 fewer reps—was 17:47. The running speed was the difference.

Next, I wanted Alex to test the final again, but another variant with a different rep scheme. Alex did a thorough warm-up, and then she was ready to start.

10-9-8 REPS OF:

HSPU ON PARALLETTES

KETTLEBELL DEADLIFTS (124 LB.)

THEN:

LUNGE 2 35-LB. KETTLEBELLS 80 FT.

On the opening set of 10, Alex did sets of 6 and 4 handstand push-ups to finish that set in 36 seconds. She broke that set of deadlifts up the same way, finishing the round in 1:10.

She broke the set of 9 handstand push-ups into 3s and finished them at 2:19. She did sets of 5 and 4 deadlifts to finish the round at 2:54.

She struggled a little on her final set of 8 handstand push-ups. She did a set of 3, rested and then kicked up for another set of 3. She hit 2 but missed the third and came off the wall. With 3 remaining, she kicked up and knocked

2 out. After a quick shakeout and rest, she did the final rep at 4:26. She ran to the 124-lb. kettlebells and did sets of 5 and 3 to finish the couplet in 4:54.

She picked up the 35-lb. kettlebells and started lunging down the floor. She got to the turnaround point at 40 feet and put them down. The Games will not have a turnaround. The athletes will just lunge the full length of the floor. Alex lunged back in one set to finish in 6:22. That's a little more than I want. I want it to be sub 6. I'll have a few more people test it, and I'll play with the rep scheme. I might even reduce it further. But I will keep the tall parallettes to make it plenty challenging.

Next, we had Paul test the Assault bike/Banger event. He warmed up and was swinging the hammer with ease and confidence. He's a large, strong dude, so I didn't think he would have much issue with this one. I asked him what his pace would be on the bike: *"Around 35 seconds?"* I suggested. He said sub 30. OK, wow. I told him Julian had done the event in 3 minutes.

### 30 CALORIES ON THE ASSAULT BIKE

### 10 FEET DOWN AND BACK ON THE BANGER

Paul cranked on the bike and finished 30 calories in 26 seconds! These guys are so strong it's mind boggling.

He picked up his hammer and started swinging it with precision and accuracy, resulting in great hits with almost every swing. He looked very composed. He made it 10 feet by 1:30, then turned around. Again, at the Games it will just be one 20-foot length with no turnaround. It's funny that this started off as 50 feet in my mind in the initial stages of planning. That's why we test these things out.

He completed the final section at 2:30, 30 seconds faster than Julian. I was impressed. As he finished, Paul was actually pretty composed compared to Julian. Paul said it was hard but not that bad. That's not what I was hoping for. His comment makes me want to increase the calories on the bike. I'm thinking 40 might be better—and it would be a good change because we used 30 at Regionals as well. I need to think about this one.

We then played some knockout and had some great rounds. I think Kelley won the most games of the six or so we played. She has a great shot for a short lady. After knockout, we sat around and I told them we were done. But it didn't feel like we were done, and they looked like they were ready for more.

I asked Kelley if she could test the interval event once more, and she said, "*Yeah.*" While she warmed up, I went into my space and started going through the schedule. I updated timing based on all the events we had tested. There will be some small tweaks throughout, but the Individual stuff is now close to complete. It's closer than it was a month or a week ago, but it's not done.

I had Kelley do a version with a grand total of 80 squats. I came up with that number because Alex had hit 70 at the 2:20 mark of her final round yesterday. I thought 80 might be a good total.

3 2-MINUTE ROUNDS AND I 3-MINUTE ROUND OF:

2 ROPE CLIMBS

7 CALORIES ON THE SKIERG

AS MANY OHS (105 LB.) AS POSSIBLE IN REMAINING TIME FOR A TOTAL OF 80 REPS

On the first round, Kelley finished the first two movements at 1:04 to Alex's 1:07. Kelley did a set of 22 overhead squats by the 2-minute mark. After Round 1, Kelley had a 2-rep lead on Alex.

On the second round, Kelley's 1:08 was slower than her first round and slower than Alex's 1:03 in Round 2. Kelley did a set of 18 unbroken squats to bring her total to 40. Alex had done 17 for 37.

On the third round, Kelley spent 1:16 getting to the bar, then did 11 squats for a total of 51. Alex took 1:08 to earn enough time for 15 reps (52 *total*). After 3 rounds, Alex had the lead by 1 rep.

On the final round, Kelley finished the first two movements in about 1:22 and had over 1:30 to finish 29 squats. It seemed like a tall task. She did a set of 14 and was at 65 by 2:30. She completed a set of 5 by 2:48, and with time running out she did 3 more for a total of 73. She was a good number short of 80 but close to 75. Alex had finished the first pairing in 1:14—almost 10 seconds faster. That allowed her to hit 70 squats by 2:20. In theory, I think she could have hit 10 more in 40 seconds. But even 5 more would have put her around 2:30, maybe even 2:35-2:40. Based on these observations and tests, I think I'll set the target at 75 for the next test. That's probably the sweet spot. Next week, I'll have Julian test this with 75.

And that was officially the end of that testing block. We had a great few days that produced lots of good data for me to work with. I took them to lunch, and Kelley dug into a stack of gluten-free pancakes. Paul had fried chicken and waffles. Alex kept her lunch clean.

I'm done with them here. I'll see them in about a month at the Games, where they will also test a handful of events.

Even though they are leaving, testing continues tomorrow and will likely go all week. It will likely continue in the week after that. I have Julian coming tomorrow at 10 a.m., and I have a big list of things for him to test before the week is out.

I'm going to hang out at Yarrow for a little longer tonight to work on some Individual items and Team stuff.

Oh, and I had another really good idea for the 2018 Games, which I can't talk about here.

*Monday, July 3, 12:19 p.m.*
Today I had Matt and Julian both come for testing. I decided to have Matt test the GGGMW chipper.

80 PULL-UPS

70 GHD SIT-UPS

60 PISTOLS

40 CALORIES ON THE CONCEPT2 ROWER

20 PUSH PRESSES (100-LB. DUMBBELL, SWITCHING ARMS EVERY 5 REPS)

This one isn't very technical. Matt quickly warmed up and attacked it. He started off with a set of 40 pull-ups, then broke the rest into 10s or so until he hit 80. Both Paul and Kelley had finished this portion in 1:30. Matt was a little over 2 minutes.

He started grinding through GHD reps, and he was much slower than I expected. He broke them up a handful of times, and he was also only using one hand to touch the ground. *(After testing, I asked him what was up. It turned out he had done a lot of GHDs yesterday.)*

In the pistols, he instantly felt the fatigue from the other sections, specifically the 70 GHD reps. The GHD-pistol combo had caused Paul to miss some pistols in the beginning, and it caused some problems for Matt, too. They both struggled on the first 10 or so. The pistols took Matt about 4 minutes to finish.

As Matt was walking over to row, Stephane said, "*OK, now you can recover on the row.*"

"*Bullshit!*" I yelled. "*Go hard!*"

After getting off the rower, Matt was severely gassed. I think he waited almost a minute before picking up the dumbbell. He did his first 10 unbroken, then did 5 and 5. His total time was 14:58, about 1:30 slower than Paul. Paul and Matt are at very different levels, but it was a very good performance by Matt. I'll probably have another person test it soon.

Next, we played some knockout—which has become a mandatory part of the warm-up process for Julian. I think he uses it more for the mental warm-up than the physical. Julian actually doesn't warm up that much. He's usually ready to go right away. I let him know that he was going to do the interval test. His target goal would be 75 OHS. We've done a few versions already, and it seems 75 might be the right number.

3 2-MINUTE ROUNDS AND 1 3-MINUTE ROUND OF:

2 ROPE CLIMBS

10 CALORIES ON THE SKIERG

AS MANY OHS (155 LB.) AS POSSIBLE IN REMAINING TIME FOR A TOTAL OF 75 REPS

Julian's first round went great. He was done with the first two parts in 1 minute, and he did 20 OHS. He actually had about 8 seconds left, and he just stopped and rested.

On his second round, he did 2 rope climbs in 16 seconds—4 seconds faster than his first round—and finished the calories at 59 seconds. He got 20 squats.

On his third round, he did the climbs in 18 seconds and came off the SkiErg at 1:02 before doing 18 OHS to take his total to 58.

He had to do 17 reps in the final round, and he had an extra minute to work with. Julian once again completed his rope climbs in about 19 seconds, and he finished the 10 calories at 1:07. It was his slowest round, as you would expect. He then picked up the bar and hit about 69 squats around the 2-minute mark. He finished all 75 at 2:06.

I was impressed. He crushed it. He would have made it even with 80.

A couple of things to consider: Julian considers overhead squats a strength, and he's fresh and rested. He's also done variants of this event a few times, so he knows what to expect from it and how to game it. This will be one of the last events at the Games—second to last actually—so the athletes should have some fatigue kicking in.

As we were chatting it up, I was thinking about who else can test it. Dynamis CrossFit is about 3 miles from Yarrow and had a young guy qualify for Regionals this year. While Julian recovered, I texted Connor Cackovic to ask him if he could test this week. He said yes, and then I followed up with this: *"Can you test in a few hours?"* He said yes. Good answer. So he's in the gym warming up as I type this.

I asked him if he is a good overhead squatter, and he said yes. Another good answer. I explained the event to him and told him his target is 75 reps. I didn't tell him what Julian got or that anyone else had done it. I want him to figure a plan out on his own and tackle this with no knowledge of what's possible.

*1:48 p.m.*
Just had Connor go through the test. He was 23rd in the California Regional, so he's a great athlete but not a top competitor like Julian or Paul, guys who have been to the Games. In Julian's case, he actually qualified for the Games this year. The difference between Connor and Julian is huge. It's the same as the difference between Matt and Julian. As good as Matt is in testing events for me, I still need top guys to get a real sense of what's possible with Games events.

3 2-MINUTE ROUNDS AND 1 3-MINUTE ROUND OF:

2 ROPE CLIMBS

10 CALORIES ON THE SKIERG

AS MANY OHS (155 LB.) AS POSSIBLE IN REMAINING TIME FOR A TOTAL OF 75 REPS

Connor started off great. He did 2 rope climbs in 23 seconds and finished the first pairing in 59 seconds—faster than Julian. He did a big set of 20 unbroken squats and had a few seconds remaining, but he used them for extra rest.

On his second round, he finished the first pairing in 1:05, then got 10 squats before putting the bar down. In the remaining time, he got 4 more. So his total was 34. This is where you see the difference between guys like Julian and Connor. At this stage, Julian was up to 40 via 2 unbroken sets of 20 in a row.

On his third round, Connor did 6 overhead squats before dropping, bringing his total to 40. He did 7 more for 47. At this stage Julian was at 58.

To finish, Connor needed 28 OHS in the final round. It seemed like a tall task but I was interested to see how it went. Connor finished 2 rope climbs in 30 seconds and was off the SkiErg by 1:20. He walked over to the bar and got 10 squats before dropping the bar at the 2-minute mark with 57 total. In Julian's test, he had finished 75 at 2:06. Connor had 1 minute remaining. He got 3 more for a total of 60, dropped the bar, rested and then squeaked out 5 more for a total of 65.

Having seen two athletes of different abilities do this event, I now believe 75 might be more appropriate than 80. I figure no athlete will finish 25 in each of the first 3 rounds to complete 75 total. I think that's very unlikely. Julian did 20-20-18 for 58 in 3 rounds. Using 75 will make it come down to the number of reps an athlete has to do in the final round. Julian had 17, and he did that in one set. Connor had 28, and he wasn't able to finish them in the remaining time.

We've tested this a ton, but it's necessary. The preparation and testing will ensure it's a great event. I also asked Stephane to email Jamie Hagiya and ask her if she could come test it, too. I want to see a few additional females go through it now.

*6:39 p.m.*

This evening I went to Yarrow and worked on the schedule and Team stuff. I'm back into this place where I feel like I'm falling behind, mostly because of Team stuff and because how of much I'm testing the Individual events. I'm really trying to nail that stuff down and get it exactly where it should be. Exactly where it should be is not even defined. It's a feeling. It's when I feel it's right. And for some of the tests to get to that point, I have to keep refining them.

It's interesting. When you think of events such as the longer Amanda and heavy Amanda, I don't really test a lot. I just know they are good as is. The story they tell, the story they support is strong as is. But some of these other events—like the interval test and the final—I really need to dial them in and get them right. When I think back on it, each year I always have two or three Games events I test over and over to make sure they're exactly what I want. In 2016, I tested Rope Chipper and Redemption *(the pegboard test)* a lot. In 2015, I spent a lot of time on the pegboard event, Pedal to the Metal 1, but that was something we figured out the week of the Games through multiple iterations. I didn't have Yarrow at that time.

I feel like I made some progress tonight on Team stuff. Conceptually, when Justin suggested doing Team Amanda by gender, that helped some things fall into place. I'll have the men do 27-21-15 reps of muscle-ups and squat snatches, and then the women will go. Or maybe I'll reverse the order. Not sure yet.

That helped me figure out I have one block for a pure CrossFit-like event for the teams—meaning no Worm or other nuance. For that block, I'm going to plan an event with three mixed pairs. It will be a couplet everyone goes through, and then another couplet. The first I'm looking at is a mini chipper, probably 100 pull-ups and 100 GHD sit-ups. And then the second couplet will be something like 3 rounds of 30/20 calories and partner deadlifts. I need to play with the timing of these tests to make sure the work can be done in fewer than 20 minutes. I have a very distinct flow and layout for this that will clearly show who's winning.

Tomorrow morning, Julian, Matt and Connor will test the male section of Team Amanda. That will help me determine how much time the event will require. Then I need to spend some solo time finalizing the Team workouts. I feel like I'm in a good space right now to keep making progress on them while I continue analyzing the Individual events and figuring out the details for each one.

Some other developments going on right now include two athletes who tested positive for banned substances. One is a team member from CrossFit Marysville. Baker Leavitt from Kill Cliff is dating one of the girls from that team, Kelsey Nagel. The team has been to the Games multiple years. The person who failed the test wants to appeal. They usually do.

The second guy who failed his test is Ryan Elrod, an individual competitor from the Atlantic Regional. I remember watching him on the live stream. He's 35 or 36, I think, so it was a big deal that he qualified. Guys that old typically don't make it anymore. He was using a fertility drug that is on the banned-substance list. He wants to appeal, too. He's also trying to get to our soft side, talking about how long he and his wife have been trying to get pregnant, etc. Bottom line: The stuff he was taking is on our banned list because it is a performance-enhancing drug, whether it's for fertility or not.

They will likely both get disqualified from the Games after their appeals. This will be big news. Some drama will come from it, and I imagine the sixth-place individual and sixth-place team from those Regionals will be very upset about this. But at this stage, we can't let them in. It's too close to the event. We haven't tested them, and that's required. If we could do an "emergency" test, we wouldn't have the results back in time.

I'm also considering doing an event announcement tomorrow on the Fourth of July.

*Tuesday, July 4, 6:45 a.m.*
I had trouble sleeping last night because I was having Games dreams.

It's usually around this time every year, about a month out, that I start having dreams in which I worry about the Games and what's coming. Those dreams usually continue in different versions for a few weeks after the Games.

In last night's dream, the top women were competing in an evening event held in what seemed to be a dark version of our stadium. The test had them moving hay bales down the floor. I walked in and watched it go down. I was shirtless, and it was cold, so I asked Stephane to get me a shirt. I then walked around the perimeter of the venue, watching the event go down and taking pictures with fans. I generally walk fast and with a purpose so I won't have to take pics with fans.

Brooke Wells won this event.

*2:26 p.m.*

This morning, I met with the guys and we tested a potential Team event: Triple Amanda. Get it done however you want, with one person working at a time.

AS A TEAM OF 3, 27-21-15 REPS OF:

MUSCLE-UPS

SQUAT SNATCHES (135 LB.)

The testing crew comprised Matt, Julian and Connor—the new guy. They opted to divide up the reps equally and perform them before switching athletes. So each would do 9-9, 7-7 and 5-5. They blitzed through everything unbroken and never really looked challenged, but they were tired and it was work.

They finished the first round of muscle-ups in 1:31, spending about 30 seconds each on 9 reps. They finished the first round of snatches at 2:53.

They finished the second total round at 5:15 and the final round at 6:54. They didn't have movement or transitions like they would at the Games, but their time was faster than I expected. I don't know if this event will stay as is. I might modify it. I might not. I have to process this one a little. I also was planning on having one gender go through and then the other, but now I'm thinking of having the males do one test of it, then having the females do another separate test.

Besides that testing session, I've been trying to rest. It's Fourth of July. I hit the CrossFit.com WOD after the testing session, and it crushed me. It was a Hero Workout, Rich, and it starts with 13 snatches at 155 lb. Then you do 10 rounds of 10 pull-ups and run 100 meters. It ends with 13 squat cleans at 155. I can't do it at 155, so I scaled to 135. I started the clock, and I got a couple of reps but missed one. I kept fighting through it, but once I was in the 10s I was missing more than I was making. I looked at the clock, and it had been more than 20 minutes—and I hadn't even hit the 13th rep. I stopped the workout, reloaded the bar to 115 and tried that. It felt light, so I restarted the workout with 115-lb. snatches. I finished those in 3-something this time, and I finished the entire workout in 21 minutes. But it wore me down. I'm tired now. I'm tired today. I need a break. I need a break from it all. The Games planning is starting to catch up. Yet I know how much more I still have to do. It will all be over in a few weeks, at least for this year.

*4:52 p.m.*

I was able to gather a little motivation. I decided to announce Run Swim Run. I was going to film a little announcement, but I wasn't motivated to be in front of the camera, so I changed my mind and decided to continue the theme I used during Regionals. I filmed my announcement while writing it on a pad of paper. Technically, I wrote the Regionals announcements on a whiteboard, so a yellow pad of paper is new for the Games.

I'm glad that one is out. Now people can start wondering about the distances and details. Over the course of the next few weeks, I'll probably announce a few more. One each week or so.

*9:10 p.m.*

I just had what might be a great idea for the final. I've been using descending reps in this one—12-9-6, 10-9-8, etc. I realized I don't have any events with ascending rep schemes at this point. Here, a slightly increasing rep scheme might be very effective. Even something as low as 6-8-10 reps of parallette handstand push-ups and kettlebell deadlifts. Or 7-9-11. I like where this is going. I'll probably have Julian test this Thursday.

*Wednesday, July 5, 8:18 a.m.*

This morning I texted Connor and asked him if he could test this afternoon. He said sure. I'm going to have him test the chipper.

I also did an analysis of all the event time domains to see how long I want the chipper to be. Run Swim Run will be the longest event, over 30 minutes for most and just under 30 minutes for the fastest. We've had longer events in the past couple of years, but not much longer. Murph was a little longer at about 40 minutes. Ranch Trail Run in 2016 was over 30 minutes, and Pier Paddle in 2015 was over 40. I'm OK with not having anything longer than that this year. Longer doesn't fit, but the absence of a longer test won't change the final results or prevent us from finding the Fittest on Earth. We'll still accomplish that.

A handful of events will end up in the range of 7-11 minutes: the odd-object event, Amanda and 17.5++. Actually, the clean ladder will end up in that range for some as well.

We don't really have anything in the range of 12-15 minutes. The interval event will be in that time frame, but with rest breaks. This chipper should be a good event for that mid-range time frame.

I also wrote down what I think want to announce early. It's looking like this:

Cyclocross—but that will be more of a tease, just a pic of the bike, so people won't know if it's a mountain-bike course or what.

The 1RM snatch.

The chipper—but without the push-press weight.

The odd-object event—but without much detail.

The bar-muscle-up/clean event—without the weights.

The O-course—probably once they start building it.

The event with hay bales and 500 meters of running—again, with little detail.

That leaves the following events to be announced at the Games:

Thursday: Amanda.

Friday: Assault bike Banger.

Saturday: 17.5++.

Sunday: the interval event and the final.

As I type this, I realize we are more prepared than ever for the Individual competition at this stage. Even though I still sometimes feel like I'm rushing to get stuff done, we are in a really good place. At this stage, I'll continue to refine and tweak the events to get the exact outcome I'm looking for.

I'm currently reading *"Zen and the Art of Motorcycle Maintenance,"* and one of its central questions is, *"What is quality?"* That's exactly what I'm trying to answer for myself: What is quality in programming the Games? I'm striving for quality, and I'll know when I achieve it.

*7:53 p.m.*
Earlier today, I met up with Connor and had him test the chipper.

80 PULL-UPS

70 GHD SIT-UPS

60 PISTOLS

40 CALORIES ON THE CONCEPT2 ROWER

20 PUSH PRESSES (100-LB. DUMBBELL, SWITCHING ARMS EVERY 5 REPS)

The dumbbell really worked him over. He was doing well up until that point but took 3-4 minutes for 20 push presses. His total time was 15-something. Connor isn't a small dude, either. He's thick and strong looking. But the 100-pounder got him, especially on his left arm.

Later, I went back to Yarrow and looked over some floors Bill and his team had sent over. They're mock-ups of the rigs for the muscle-up event on Saturday and for the Sunday events. For Sunday, we need a setup for tall rope climbs and a setup for handstand push-ups. The mock-ups look good. I gave a little feedback on placement.

The muscle-up event will have four different bars, and I just decided I'll have them do the sets of 4 muscle-ups as singles. We've never done that before, and it will catch people off guard. It will end up being 36 bar muscle-ups, 4 in each round, all done as singles, and the heavy cleans. This rig will allow me some creativity with the Team programming, too. I feel like I'm really hitting a mental block with that.

Next, I forced myself to work on a Saturday Team event, and the floor mock-up with four pull-up bars in each lane really helped me. I came up with something I had already kinda built a framework around previously, but I refined it today.

In male and female pairs, they will all go through 80 pull-ups and 60 GHD sit-ups. The pull-ups will be synchronized, and they will advance to another pull-up bar every 20 reps. Then they'll do 60 synchronized GHD sit-ups. I'll have the GHDs side by side, and the rep will count when both athletes touch the top. One pair will go through everything, and then the next one goes. Once they all finish, they'll do a couplet with SkiErgs and partner deadlifts. Two rounds of it, with something like 20/16 calories.

So it would be SkiErg calories, then 18 deadlifts for the first pair, broken up into 2 sets. So they'd do 9, advance, then do another 9 to complete Round 1. Then they'd go back to the SkiErg, then back to the bar for 2 sets of deadlifts. Then the next pair goes. Maybe the next pair has to do 20 deadlifts and the final one has to do 22. Or something like that. Playing this out, I might actually change the reps on the pull-ups, too, just to provide variance and force teams to choose how they use their athletes.

The next test after that is supposed to be a Worm event, but I'm not feeling it right now. Maybe I'm just over the Worm. Maybe that's why I'm having problems programming for the teams. I feel like I need the Worm, but I don't feel the Worm. I'm way behind on Team programming, and I'm not in love with what I have right now. It feels like I'm running out of time. I'll try to dedicate next weekend to Team testing. I'll see if Stephane can line the team up for two days of testing. I really wish the teams weren't so large. It would make this process easier. The Invitational teams of four are great. Maybe we should go to that in the future.

I also worked on the plan for tomorrow's testing. I have Jamie Hagiya and Julian coming. That will make for some fun basketball. More importantly, I'm going to have Jamie try the interval event and see how the goal of 75 squats treats her. Julian is going to do the new inverted final that starts with low reps instead of higher reps. It will still end with the double-kettlebell lunges. I was playing with numbers: 7-9-11, 6-10-12. Then I thought of some of the other number patterns. I looked at triangular and square numbers, but those didn't work. Then I looked at Fibonacci numbers—and they actually work great. I found these numbers in there: 5-8-13.

In a Fibonacci sequence, every number after the first two in the pattern is the sum of the two numbers that precede it. For example, 1, 1, 2, 3, 5, 8, 13, 21—1 + 1 = 2, 1 + 2 = 3, 2 + 3 = 5, 3 + 5 = 8, 5 + 8 = 13, 8 + 13 = 21. And so on. The 5-8-13 pattern produces 26 reps, with the largest set last. I'm not sure if this will work. I want it to go fast. I think this approach will really slow the women up unless we adjust the height of the risers on the floor for the parallette HSPU. We can't make it too deep. But that's what testing is for.

For historical reference, this is not the first time I have leaned on Fibonacci sequences. I learned about it from Tony Budding one year in Carson when we were trying to figure out reps for an event we were creating.

*Thursday, July 6, 4:16 p.m.*

Matt met us at Yarrow this morning at 9 a.m. Julian was supposed to be there, too, but he always shows up 20-30 minutes late. I didn't need to wait for him and waste time, so I told Matt to warm up for the HSPU/deadlift event. This was not my original plan, but he was there and Julian wasn't. I was going to have them test the latest version with the 5-8-13 Fibonacci sequence.

Shortly before Matt began, Julian showed up, so I had him watch Matt do it. Not that that would change the results of Julian's effort, but he did have the advantage of seeing how Matt planned.

Even though they didn't do it together, I'll recount the test as if they did.

5-8-13 REPS OF:

PARALLETTE HANDSTAND PUSH-UPS

KETTLEBELL DEADLIFTS (200 LB.)

LUNGE 2 53-LB. KETTLEBELLS 80 FT.

It took Matt 11 seconds to knock out his first set of 5 handstand push-ups. Matt is strong on those. Julian took 8 seconds. They both walked over to the deadlifts, composed and controlled. Both athletes did 5 in 1 set. Matt finished at 28 seconds and Julian was done at 22.

On the second round, they both did 8 unbroken handstand push-ups, but Julian was building his lead. Julian finished 8 at 41 seconds, and Matt was done at 58 seconds. Julian, of course, did the set of 8 deadlifts unbroken. He had finished his first 2 rounds at 1:03. I was very surprised when Matt did all 8 deadlifts unbroken to finish the first 2 rounds at 1:30.

Julian stretched his lead on the final set of 13 HSPU. He did a set of 13 unbroken and finished at 1:47. Matt did 10 in 2:29, rested and then finished the last 3 at 3:04. Julian did a set of 10 deadlifts, rested briefly and then completed the final set at 2:37. Matt did 8 and 5 to finish at 4:32. Julian was almost 2 minutes ahead.

Julian lunged 40 feet, put the kettlebells down, then came back for a total time of 4:11. He was done before Matt finished his deadlifts.

On the lunges, Matt started at 4:58 and had gone 40 feet by 5:27. He turned around and went 30 feet before dropping the kettlebells. He went another 9 feet, dropping 1 foot away from the finish line. He picked them up for 1 small set and crossed the line at 6:52.

Great performances by both. But this test shows the difference between someone who is close to qualifying for Regionals and someone who has been to the Games and actually earned a spot in this year's Games.

At this point, this event is almost done. The Fibonacci sequence rounds it out nicely. And the numbers I chose—5-8-13—make it appropriately challenging.

After they were done, we had some great knockout games while we waited for Jamie. Julian was really looking forward to playing with her, but he had to leave to be back for Miranda. Jamie was not going to show up until a little later.

Once she arrived, we went right to basketball. Jamie played at USC, and she still plays. After a few rounds of knockout, I briefed her on the event. She felt ready, and she went very hard.

3 2-MINUTE ROUNDS AND 1 3-MINUTE ROUND OF:

2 ROPE CLIMBS

7 CALORIES ON THE SKIERG

AS MANY OHS (105 LB.) AS POSSIBLE IN REMAINING TIME FOR A TOTAL OF 75 REPS

She crushed the first 2 rope climbs, finishing in 18 seconds. That's comparable to what the guys did on that section. Then she absolutely murdered the SkiErg, finishing at 49 seconds. None of the others had finished that fast—not even the men.

She started cranking on the overhead squats, and I thought she was going to stop at 15 reps. She muscled out 20, and I was convinced she was going to put it down. But she kept going and got 25. Her form is great in that movement, but it looked like she was fighting for the reps, especially in the 15-25 range. Her total was greater than anyone else's in the first round. Stephane and I were blown away. She finished 25 on her first round, leaving

50 for the next 3 rounds, including the final round with an additional minute to work. Apparently 75 reps would not be an issue.

After her 1-minute rest, she attacked Round 2, which caught her by surprise. She finished the rope climbs in 27 seconds, almost 10 seconds slower than Round 1, and she was off the SkiErg at 1:06, almost 20 seconds off her Round 1 pace. She walked to the bar, labored to get it up and then knocked out a set of 8. She was able to get it up again for 7 more reps. She got 15 total reps for a 2-round total of 40—still a good place to be.

She slowed further on Round 3. She finished the first two movements at 1:18. When she walked over to the chalk bucket, I shot a worried glance at Stephane. The clock was ticking. She was able to get 10 squats, bringing her total to 50. At this point, Julian had done 58.

We told Jamie she had to do 25 in her final round, and she understood. She finished the rope climbs and SkiErg at 1:27, and she was close to 1:50 by the time she got to the bar, set up and snatched it. She did a couple of big sets and was able to get to 60 with about 30 seconds remaining. She grabbed the bar and fought to get a few more squats, and she finished with 66 reps. She didn't hit 75 but actually wasn't too far away.

She had put in a strong effort and really enjoyed the event. She said it hurt and that her gas isn't where it should be right now because she's focusing more on getting strong. But she believed the test is appropriate for the girls at the Games. I believe it is, too. I would like to get one more female to test it—and hopefully complete it. Julian completed 75 by the 2:11 mark of the final round, but he's great at overhead squats.

I'm really happy with this one and where it's ended up after all the testing and planning. Not much will change now. I feel like we're almost there with the Individual events. I'll do a little more testing and tweaking, but they're pretty close.

I'm still at Yarrow, so I'm going to work on the Team events. I have a pair of athletes coming tomorrow to test a pairs event I came up with.

*Friday, July 7, 2:30 p.m.*
On a flight right to HQ with Mike on our plane. I have Zoë with me. I'm taking her to see her grandmother. It's Finley's birthday tomorrow, and she's having a sleepover. Sage and I decided it would be best if Zoë and I went

away for the weekend so Fin could have her birthday party and sleepover with just her friends. Zoë is at the age where she is really not into the things Finley is into, and it's easiest if they are separate for events like sleepovers.

We're going to drop her off in Oakland, where she will be picked up by Carlanne, her grandmother. Then Mike is taking me up to Santa Rosa, where I will Uber over to Satya Kraus' motorcycle shop and pick up my Harley-Davidson Road Glide. Satya did a bunch of custom work to it, and I haven't seen it in months. I'm very excited about reuniting with the bike.

After that, I'll drive to Santa Cruz. The work part of this trip is a speaking engagement I have as part of a Stanford business program for vets. Stanford runs a multi-week summer program for vets who recently got out and are getting into the business world. Someone from the program asked if I would speak, and I thought it would be a good opportunity to give back. But this is the only date they had, right in the middle of Games season. When I agreed to it, I wasn't thinking about the timing. In the past few weeks, I've gone through various stages of wanting to pull out to being OK with it. The event is less than 24 hours away, and I'm comfortable now, maybe even a little excited.

I'm going to tell my story, and CrossFit's, and explain how I got to this point. Along the way, I have some suggestions and advice. Organizing my thoughts usually helps me overcome my fears with events like this. What really puts me at ease is the fact that we'll open up with a group workout. That's a great way to get everyone to loosen up. I also look forward to meeting everyone and hearing about their time in the military. After I finish this entry, I'll start scripting my talk in detail. Writing this book has helped me learn to type and organize my thoughts very well.

I'm traveling today, but testing didn't stop. This morning at 8 a.m., I had a pair of athletes show up to test a Team event. Connor came, as well as Kendall Morris, the strong female from CrossFit Forest.

I had them start with 80 pull-ups and 60 GHD sit-ups—both synchronized. It didn't start off great. To my surprise, Kendall needed to break up the reps right away. I'm talking sets of less than 10. I was really surprised. So around the 45-rep mark, I called an audible and told them to do 62 instead. This is OK because one of the versions would have that low number. They then did the 60 sit-ups, and it actually looked like Connor struggled a little and slowed them up. They finished that couplet in about 5 or so minutes, and I had them rest 7 minutes before starting the second piece.

In theory, the other two pairs will get their work done during that rest. But the couplet shouldn't have taken so long. I'll have to scale the reps a little to speed it up.

The second part was 2 rounds of 20/16 calories on the SkiErg and 20 heavy partner deadlifts. We used 5 reds—55 lb. each—on one side and 5 blues (*45 lb. each*) on the other. Connor crushed the calories, and then on Round 1 they did a set of 10 deadlifts. That crushed them. The next set of 10 was really slow. On the second round, Kendall actually came off the bike first, reminiscent of how she crushed the rower in previous testing with her team. I knew a set of 20 was going to be very difficult, so I dropped the reps to 16. They ended up doing that in 3 sets, but it was still very difficult. It's over programmed for what I need it to be. I need to take this one back to the drawing board. Not the concept, but the reps and amount of work. I tasked Stephane with looking into how it could fit in our timeline. I'll see what he comes back with.

On this little road trip, I plan on taking a little break from programming today and tomorrow. I'll dive back in Sunday when we get home. But for the next two days, I'll leave it. I probably won't stop thinking about it, but I won't sit down and do specific work on it. Should be a nice little forced reset period for me.

*Saturday, July 8, 1:48 p.m.*
The previous two days have gone well. I picked up my motorcycle from Satya Kraus, and it looks amazing. I couldn't believe how well it came out. While waiting for him to finish it, we took a little trip over to visit CrossFit NorthGate, the affiliate he trains at. That was fun. I really enjoy getting into the community and visiting boxes during my travels. It's great to see the varying levels of people who train at the affiliates. My world, for the most part, is filled with CrossFit Games athletes, but they are not representative of the type of client you run into at a typical CrossFit affiliate. And that's a good thing. Most people are at CrossFit gyms to make changes in their lives and improve their health, whereas the Games athletes are trying to maximize their performance. Two different goals, same program.

After the visit, I went back to Satya's motorcycle shop. We just hung out and looked at the bikes, talked bikes. It was great to clear my mind of the Games grind.

Once the bike was ready, we discussed how I should get back to Santa Cruz. Satya advised taking the 101 across the Golden Gate and the 1 all the way down. I contemplated that but thought maybe I should just get back. But then I thought, *"Here I am with this badass bike and some time for a minor reset and rest from the Games stuff. How often will I have that bike and this opportunity?"* So I went for it.

I left his place around 7 and crossed the Golden Gate to hit the 1 and head south. It was a great ride, great scenery. It was nice to zone out and just enjoy crossing beautiful landscape. The road and the ride reminded me of a couple of books I have read, most recently *"Zen and the Art of Motorcycle Maintenance"* and Hunter S. Thompson's *"Hell's Angels."* There is one part in the book where Thompson is hauling ass down the 1 in stiff rain and cold at night and he feels like he's going to die. My ride reminded me of that, though I was not driving too fast and I didn't feel like I was going to die—but it was cold, and I was not prepared. Inland all across the Bay it was around 90 F or more, so I wasn't expecting the coast to be so cool. I should have known better.

This morning, I met with the group from the Stanford Ignite program, and we did a little workout, something very similar to what we did in Madison a few weeks ago. It was a team workout that involves synchronized movement, coordination and communication within teams of four. I learned today that teams of three work perfectly in this format, too. This is a keeper for other events. I'll for sure refer back to it in the future.

After the workout, I gave a presentation and talked for a few hours. They were a great group and seemed to enjoy it. They all had positive things to say, but I think I was kind of off. I could have done better. I think this was simply a rehearsal I can improve on. I hope to have the chance to work with this group again and do more stuff with individuals like this.

I'm back in my hotel room contemplating what to do. I might take a nap and then go for a nice long ride on the new bike. Maybe go to The Ranch and see my dad, check the place out. Possibly just cruise around the area and relax.

I'm happy with how these two days are playing out. Tomorrow, I go back to Games mode to finalize the last pieces. I'm excited about the Games. They're going to be the best yet. I have no doubt about that.

*Sunday, July 9, 9:37 a.m.*

Heading home today from Santa Cruz. I have to be back up here again on Wednesday for another HQ meeting. But rather than stay for the three days in between, it's important for me to get back to testing so I can finalize more of the programming. I have Lindsey Valenzuela coming to Yarrow tomorrow. I'm going to have her test the interval event. We haven't had a female finish it yet. Alex was close, but she didn't have the target of 75 in mind. Kelley and Jamie both missed it. I think Lindsey will be a good one to test it. She's a fighter, she's strong, and she moves well, so this plays to her strengths.

Before leaving I had breakfast with Sevan and Justin. We went over some of the details of the upcoming Games, and I shared a couple of big-picture ideas for next year's Games. I can't outline them here for obvious reasons, but they are floating around and will need a lot of involvement to pull off, so we need to start planting the seeds now. I say this quite often, but I really do plan various stages of these events years out. I'm finalizing this year's programming but haunted by ideas I think will be amazing in next year's Games. It's a great feeling to know I've made progress in planning 2018 before the 2017 Games start.

*4:53 p.m.*

I've been home for a few hours. I was going to try to take a nap, but I couldn't get into it. My mind isn't settled, and I still feel like I have a lot to do—which is accurate. I came down to my home office and did some seminar work. I caught up on that standard work, talked to Sevan and Nicole, and got up to speed on some big-picture CrossFit things from the past few days.

After that, I opened up a drive folder with the floor layouts I created a few days ago. I had Stephane populate it with the current floors for the Individual events. These are the mock-ups, the CAD drawings, for every event we will do at the Games on our standard floors. I expected to see one or two, but he had done them all for the Coliseum events. That's the majority of the events. All the floors for all four days of competition are in that folder, and I went through each to offer feedback. This turned the juices back on and made me excited. Seeing them all done and knowing they are all basically there is exciting. We have floors and signage already being created, and that has to be a record for us in the 11 years of the Games. This has given me some momentum, and I might go to Yarrow and work on Team programming now.

*Monday, July 10, 8:10 p.m.*
I didn't go to Yarrow last night.

On Friday as I was getting ready to travel up to Santa Cruz, I saw that we had a Masters specialty course in San Diego this weekend. Chuck Carswell, one of our senior Seminar Staff members and head judge for the Games' Team competition *(with Todd Widman)* teaches that course. I asked if he could stay until Monday so we could meet. He agreed, and Mallee Sato changed his travel to accommodate.

We met at 9 a.m. this morning and went through all the Team events day by day. Starting with Run Swim Run, we decided whether each pair would hold a short rope. We agreed to include the rope. Then we went to the Team Amanda event. I had some new rep schemes sketched out on the board, and we agreed to use those, with more reps for the male trio than the female trio.

We saw no issues with the O-course. We know we need to figure the timing and everything else out on site to determine what the event will look like. It doesn't make sense to program when we haven't even seen the final product.

We also worked through the flow and timing of the 1RM squat clean and jerk, and we finalized the reps of the row/Worm-squat event: 3 rounds of 40/30 calories and 30 squats.

Then we looked at Saturday's events. The day opens with the Big Bob. We decided we can't do much with that until we can test it on the actual field with the actual Big Bobs. But we have an idea of how long the test should be.

Then we dove into the two Saturday-afternoon tests that are not done. I had one tested recently but not the other. I tasked Chuck with figuring out some rep schemes for the concepts I had, and he dove into that after we were done with all the other days. He had an interesting idea that I liked and will allow. One event is a pairs relay with two couplets. So one pair does one couplet, and when they finish, the second pair goes through, followed by the third pair. Then they move through another couplet test. My original plan was to use mixed pairs throughout, but Chuck suggested allowing teams to do whatever they want for the first couplet. Here's why that makes sense: The first couplet is going to be 24 muscle-ups and 50 GHD sit-ups, with variations requiring 20 and 16 bar muscle-ups. So in theory you could put your top two guys together for the version with 24, then have a male and female on the 20-50 version, followed by a pair of females on the 16-50 version. But when you come to the next couplet, it will have to be mixed pairs throughout.

For the final event Saturday, I laid out the concept and then Chuck plugged in reps and rounds. He was thinking 2 rounds of pull-ups, toes-to-bars, Assault bike calories and Worm cleans. I like his version. Originally, I was thinking 3 rounds.

Ah, I just saw a problem with that. I'll have to revisit it with him. Basically, 3 rounds ensured that everyone hit each station: pull-ups, toes-to-bars and bike. That won't happen with 2 rounds—unless I'm missing something.

Oh, maybe he has 2 rounds for Sunday's test. Probably. I don't have the notes in front of me for those events as I make this entry.

The Sunday-morning Worm-run event is likely going to stay the same, but we'll test it so we have some times to play around with. After that event, we're going to cut to 20 teams so we'll have two heats of 10 for the final test, which has rope climbs and handstand push-ups with Worm work—a lot of Worm work. This one will be good. I need to test it and see if it has the bite I want.

While all this was going on, Lindsey showed up. She's a great competitor I've known for a long time, and she's an equally great person. I've always liked the fire she breathes when she takes the competition floor. She leaves it all out there. I was excited for her to tackle the interval event. If anyone in the testing pool of women could finish it, I knew she could.

I briefed her on the whiteboard. By the time I was done, she was as excited as I was. She had some questions about the requirements and flow but felt confident she could hit 75. She began a short warm-up routine.

3 2-MINUTE ROUNDS AND 1 3-MINUTE ROUND OF:

2 ROPE CLIMBS

7 CALORIES ON THE SKIERG

AS MANY OHS (105 LB.) AS POSSIBLE IN REMAINING TIME FOR A TOTAL OF 75 REPS

She attacked Round 1 like a champ. Her first two rope climbs were done in 19 seconds—equal to the times of our fastest males. She hit the SkiErg hard and ripped off 7 calories to finish at 45 seconds. *(Prior to the test, she had mentioned she used the SkiErg a ton during pregnancy, so she's very comfortable with it.)* She used a squat snatch for the first rep, than proceeded to crank out a set of 22. She dropped the bar at 1:42 and decided to rest for the remaining time. Great round.

Her Round 2 rope climbs were almost as fast as her Round 1 climbs. She finished them in 20 seconds. Her pace on the SkiErg almost matched that of the previous round, too. She finished that at 48 seconds. She walked over to the bar, took a breath, picked it up and knocked out 16 reps to take her total to 38. She put the bar down at 1:50. I think she should have squeaked out a few more reps in both rounds. She should have put it down when she did and then used a power snatch to set up a few more reps before time expired. Then again, perhaps that plan would have really slowed the next rounds. I doubt it, but it's possible.

Her Round 3 rope climbs were her slowest. She finished them at 26 seconds, and she was off the SkiErg at 1:00. She squatted 12 reps for a total of 50, stopping around 1:50. Again, I don't think this is the best strategy. I think on a test like this you need to squeak out extra reps with all the time you have. At this stage, she had finished 50 reps, with 25 remaining. Because she had stopped early in each round, she had left 38 seconds on the table in the previous rounds. That's a lot of time for reps. I doubted she could hit 75, even with the extra minute in the final round.

Even though I really doubted Lindsey, I encouraged her before the final round. She came in at an aggressive pace and finished the two rope climbs in 23 seconds. She was done with the SkiErg at 1:00 and was in much better position than Jamie was. Jamie had finished the SkiErg at 1:27, and she didn't start squatting until 1:50, leaving 9 reps incomplete when time expired. Lindsey snatched the bar overhead and got 12 reps before dropping it at 1:50. With 62 total, she had about 1:10 for 13 reps more. I was convinced she wouldn't finish. She rested, looked at the clock and got back under the bar. She had squeezed out 9 more by 2:45, then dropped the bar. We were screaming at her. After a very short rest, she ripped off the last 4 at lightning pace to finish her 75th at 2:54—6 seconds under the time cap.

I was wrong, and I was impressed. But that's why we brought her down. We had hoped she would be the female tester who could finish it.

Afterward, we chatted about the test. She really liked it. She believes it's appropriate for the top ladies and thinks it will make a great race. I'm happy now that I've seen her do it. I think it's pretty much set. I don't know if I'll have anyone test it again. Maybe I'll have a few Demo Team members go through it in Madison if we get bored.

We hung out for a bit, and then I asked if she wanted to test one more. She said, "*Sure,*" so I briefed her on the final. It was not my intention to have her test both events. I hadn't even thought to do it. But after seeing her recover, it made sense. I've not had a female try the new Fibonacci test.

I briefed her on the event: 5-8-13 parallette HSPU and deadlifts with the 124-lb. kettlebells, then 80 feet of overhead walking lunges. She started preparing while I went to the whiteboard with Stephane. In the Fibonacci sequence, 3 comes before 5—3-5-8-13. Given the height of the parallettes, I honestly think 5-8-13 might be too aggressive to create the speed I want. Because Lindsey had done a very hard event about 30 minutes prior, I decided to have her do a shorter version. Right before she started, I told her to do 3-5-8 instead. Something else I figured out: 89 comes later in the Fibonnaci sequence. Perfect. I'll make the final lunges 89 feet. That way all the reps and distances in this workout are from the Fibonacci sequence. Cool.

Lindsey finished 3 HSPU unbroken in 10 seconds, then finished 3 deadlifts at 20 seconds. Her 5 HSPU were done at 37 seconds, and the deadlifts were done at 53 seconds. Maybe this was too easy—but remember I'm trying to have athletes finish under 6 minutes.

Lindsey did 3 HSPU and came off the wall at 1:13. She did another pair, then kicked up and squeaked out 2 more. She finished her final one at 2:03, so that round of 8 was tough for her. She broke the deadlifts into 2 sets and finished them at 2:35. That's a little fast, but I believe the 5-8-13 version would have put her well off the pace I want. I'll test this one again, probably with the Demo Team. I know now the workout will use one of these two variations. About 20 seconds after finishing the first couplet, Lindsey picked up the kettlebells and lunged 40 feet. She put them down for less than 15 seconds, then lunged 40 feet back to finish at 3:56.

Something to remember: The paralletes they use at the Games will be about 4 inches higher than the ones at Yarrow. That will make a big difference. This version might be spot on.

The rest of my afternoon was hectic. I didn't dedicate the time and effort I wanted to working on the programming, but I'll dive in tomorrow, when I have more time. And, of course, we will test tomorrow.

*Tuesday, July 11, 12:43 p.m.*

This morning I had Matt and Connor meet at 10 a.m. to test the Saturday Team event that features a pair of couplets for each pair. The first couplet is 24 bar muscle-ups and 50 GHD sit-ups. In the original version we tested *(with Connor)*, we used pull-ups instead of muscle-ups. Teams will have three versions of the couplet: 24 and 50, 20 and 50, and 16 and 50 reps. The teams can use any pair of individuals for each. Again, this was Chuck's idea.

I had Connor and Matt test 24 and 50, as it's likely all teams will use a male pair here unless they have a female who is very strong at bar muscle-ups relative to the men on the team. They had to do the bar muscle-ups at four different stations—4 sets of 6.

## 24 BAR MUSCLE-UPS IN SETS OF 6

## 50 GHD SIT-UPS

The first 6 took about 18 seconds, the second set was complete at 40 seconds, and the third set was finished at 1:05—all unbroken. They took a short break before doing the final set of 6 unbroken. The last set looked a little more labored. They finished it at 1:35.

They started the GHD sit-ups at 1:45 and had finished 25 by 2:45. The second 25 took another minute. They got off the GHDs at 3:47.

I let them rest until the 12-minute mark, simulating the time it would take for the other pairs to do their work. Then Matt and Connor started this:

## 2 ROUNDS OF:

## 16 CALORIES ON THE ASSAULT BIKE

## 16 PARTNER DEADLIFTS (595 LB.)

In Round 1, they both finished the calories in about 38 seconds. According to plan, they started strong, then coasted. They did 8 deadlifts, moved the bar forward, then did 8 more to finish at 1:42. The reps looked tough, and they worked hard to get sets of 8.

They went back to the Assault bikes, and both took over a minute to finish the calories. They went to the bar and did a set of 8, moved the bar, did a set of 5, dropped it, then finished with a set of 3. They both collapsed on the floor in agony, rolling and moaning. It lit them up.

It had taken almost 5 minutes, so about 15 minutes for all pairs. If I guess that the first couplet will take 3:30 or so per pair, that's 10:30. Add in 15 minutes for the second couplet, and they'll need 25:30 to finish. I have this booked as a 21-minute heat, so I need to do one of two things: Drastically reduce the reps on the second couplet or increase the time cap.

Once Matt and Connor had recovered, we talked about some good options to reduce the reps but keep them very challenging. I'll take a close look at this one this afternoon and make a decision on the direction it will go.

*Wednesday, July 12, 7:18 p.m.*
Once again, I'm on our plane for another meeting of HQ department heads. I was going to try to get out of this meeting because of the Games and the programming crunch I feel I'm up against. But as I think through our progress, I feel confident in stepping away for a couple of days.

Even though I was just up in Scotts Valley a few days ago, I needed to come home rather than stay there for this meeting. I came home to reset, to stay with my family and to program. I hate that this meeting is scheduled right now. I think it could have waited until after the Games, but the Games are not the only thing in the company, so I realize how important the meeting is.

Greg is going to present to us. He's supposed to sit through our meetings and the presentations we are to make, and at 1 he's scheduled to give a presentation to all HQ employees in the office. Afterward, a taco truck will come by for lunch, and people will hang out. I'll bolt as soon as I can.

My Road Glide is at Sevan's house because Tyson Oldroyd had to replace the pipe on it. I'll ride that home tomorrow after the meeting. It's a long ride—probably six or seven hours—but it will clear my mind. I enjoy the coast, and it will be great to finally get the Road Glide back home. I love that bike, and I can't wait to put some serious miles on it.

I should be able to make the trip home in one day, but I might get home late Thursday night. If it gets too late or I get too tired, I'll just stop and get a hotel, probably in Santa Barbara or North L.A. Maybe even Beverly Hills. But not before that.

We don't have any testing scheduled on Friday. Stephane is actually flying to the office with me. He needs to meet with Wilson Tang to go over the schedule, and he probably won't get back until Friday afternoon anyway. But we'll see. I've often just woken up and decided to call someone over to test.

No testing Saturday, either. I'll probably spend Saturday refining the last few Team events that we'll test on Sunday. Sunday is a big day: We have Paradiso CrossFit coming down. The group finished seventh at the California Regional.

Today I also looked at a calendar and realized I still have another weekend at home before I leave for the Games. So I might have a team test then, too.

I feel like the Individual events are mostly done at this point. I need to take a day or two—probably Monday or Tuesday—to just analyze everything. I'll perform what I consider a global look to see all the parts in relation to the others. I might see some trends I don't like or will accept. I have to see all this before I finalize things. But you never know—I could change some things up. We still have time to change minor things, not for the sake of changing but to increase the quality.

Back to what we did today. I met the crew at 10 a.m.: Matt, Connor and Julian. I recently received the Slaters farmers-carry handles, so I decided to test that event to narrow down the loads.

Honestly, I showed up to testing and didn't feel like doing any of it. I felt over it. I felt like just saying, *"Hey, we don't need to test. Sorry. Just go home."* I need some alone time to work and get my thoughts organized. It's been a long week, especially at home, and I think some of it was just catching up to me.

I sat down on some Rogue risers and asked Stephane if we should test the handstand-walk event.

*"Fuck, yeah!"* he replied.

His enthusiastic response energized me. It was the boost I needed.

I told the guys to set it up, and we spent the next 15-20 minutes loading and briefing. Matt knew most of the plan already because he had been in one of my discussions with Stephane about a month back. He understood the concept.

I quickly scanned through and decided to have Matt go first. We could make adjustments after that test. Then Connor would go, allowing us to make more adjustments. Then Julian could test the corrected version.

Prior to starting, we played our mandatory knockout rounds. I was off. I don't think I won any games today. I need to win more and more consistently. I'll keep practicing and keep shooting.

For Matt, we set up the handles at 175 lb. a side, and we loaded the yoke and sled with 4 55-lb. plates each.

2 ROUNDS OF:

CARRY 3 OBJECTS 90 FT. (YOKE, SLED, FARMERS HANDLES)

ONCE EACH OBJECT IS ON OTHER SIDE, HANDSTAND WALK BACK TO START

To start, Matt carried the handles 90 feet in 16 seconds, and it took him about 1:15 to finish the first handstand walk. He decided to pull the sled next, and that took him about 30 seconds. He completed the second handstand walk at 3:45. He got the yoke down at 4:24, then chose to move the handles back first. That was fast. He was done with the handles at 4:45.

The third handstand walk started to eat him up, and we realized the ground was burning his hands. He finished walking at 7:37, then pulled the sled all the way back at 7:50. I said he could stop, but he wanted to finish. It looked like his hands were killing him, but he fought through it to finish the final handstand walk at 10:37. He brought the yoke back and completed the event at 11:07.

Some changes needed to be made. We couldn't have Julian do that version, even though he said he really wanted to and could do it outside. We told him to just run back and do his handstand walks inside. We also decided to add more weight to the handles.

Julian's test went much better than Matt's, even with additional time spent running inside to do the handstand walking. He moved the farmers handles first and finished the first handstand walk at 1:24. The weight on the handles looked much more appropriate. He chose the sled next, and he was done with that and the second handstand walk at 3:12. I think he put the yoke down once, and he was done with it by 3:41.

Julian chose to take the sled back first, and that took him about a minute. His third handstand walk took a little under a minute. He finished that section at 5:38. He moved the yoke next and finished at 6:25. His final handstand walk took less than a minute, and he finished at 7:22. He carried the handles home and stopped the clock at 7:56—which is all great considering he had to move an additional 360 feet to get back inside to perform each handstand walk.

At this point, there was no reason to have Connor try it. We can wait until Madison to test it again. We need to see how the field affects the sled.

I told Connor to warm up for squat snatches and muscle-ups. He was going to test the plussed-up version of Amanda. As he was warming up, Julian asked me why I'm testing it again. I just said it's part of the process. We test and we test some more. We rehearse and we rehearse some more. I guess those words are almost interchangeable. We're testing events for the CrossFit Games, but we're also rehearsing the execution of the CrossFit Games. Often, one rehearsal, one test, is not enough.

I didn't know how Connor would do on this test. I was kind of indifferent to it. I wanted him to do it to provide some additional data points, but I didn't really have any specific expectations for him. He's a good athlete who finished 23rd at Regionals. But Julian is a great athlete who qualified for the Games. When Julian did this test, I didn't think he did a great job, and I later learned that he agreed with me. Apparently he had done a monster squat workout the day before and was very sore from that. But he fought through and put up 12:07 on the first test of this Amanda variation.

13-11-9-7-5 REPS OF:

RING MUSCLE-UPS

SQUAT SNATCHES

Connor finished the first 13 muscle-ups in 52 seconds. Julian's split time *(from his June 3 test)* was slightly slower: 54 seconds. Connor did all his snatches in singles, whereas Julian had used 3 sets. Connor's first round was complete at 2:19 to Julian's 2:00.

On the next round, Connor finished the 11 muscle-ups at 3:30 and the snatches at 4:50. Julian had finished this round at 4:36, so Connor was behind.

On the set of 9 muscle-ups, Connor was pretty consistent and finished at 5:54. He singled his snatches and finished the round at 7:12. I don't remember exactly what happened to Julian on this round, but the muscle-ups must have slowed him because he finished at 7:13. His 14-second lead had become a 1-second deficit.

Connor was solid for sets of 4 and 3 muscle-ups, and then he continued with 7 snatch singles. His split was 9:34 to Julian's 10:32.

Connor finished 1 set of 5 muscle-ups at 10:31. He fought through the snatches and actually threw in a few touch-and-go reps to finish at 11:00. Julian's time was 12:09. Julian was sitting right next to me as Connor worked, and I could tell he was not super excited. I imagine he'll try the workout again on his own just to beat Connor's time. I love seeing that the top guys are super competitive. They should be. Don't come out and compete unless you want to kick ass and take names.

It was a good day of testing even though I wasn't into it at first. We're about to land in Watsonville, so I'm going to log off. I might not write another entry until Friday or Saturday, depending on how my trip south on the Harley goes.

*Thursday, July 13, 5:53 a.m.*
I was dreaming about the rep scheme for the final event—the Fibonacci sequence for parallette handstand push-ups and deadlifts. I woke up doubting my current plan. Maybe I need to increase the numbers, and maybe I need to ditch the Fibonacci sequence and just go 6-7-8 or something like that for the women.

Now that I'm thinking about it, I'm less worried that the current version is poor. I think it's a good version, but we'll test it again when we get to Madison to collect some more data.

Actually, scratch that. I looked at a calendar, and we still have two weeks here in California. I need to do more testing now. I just texted Bill and asked him to ship me some of the actual parallettes we'll use at the Games. That's been one of the problems with testing: We don't have the right parallettes. I'll get that corrected and do more testing here. I need to if I'm having dreams about problems with the rep scheme.

*Friday, July 14, 7:26 p.m.*

I had a long ride home yesterday. I thought it would be quick considering I can do the drive solo in seven hours, sometimes high sixes. I figured on the bike I would have no problem getting home in seven, but traffic was thick within five minutes of leaving the Scotts Valley office. I hit heavy traffic in Santa Cruz, and that slowed me up considerably. I decided to head down the 101 and rode 120 miles or so before stopping for gas in Paso Robles. The stop was necessary because my ass was on fire, too. I got back on the freeway and hit more traffic about 30 minutes later in Pismo. I didn't expect that traffic, either, and it slowed the trip even more. I made one more quick stop south of Ventura for gas and a burger, then hit the road for the final 150 miles.

Getting through Calabasas and that portion of the 101 was good—it's usually hit or miss with traffic. I exited onto the 405 for the final long stretch home and hit a ton of traffic at 9 at night. There's always traffic in L.A. Always. Doesn't matter what time of the day. Even in the middle of night, you end up hitting traffic in the most unexpected places. I ended up getting home at 10:40—eight hours on the road. I'm not happy about how long it took, but I'm happy to be home.

Today I was a bit out of my routine, so I worked out and did some routine CrossFit work. I also took care of my standard catch-up errands. This evening I decided to come to Yarrow, and I've been here for about an hour or so, just analyzing the Individual events to look for patterns—or a lack of patterns. I updated the list of all the movements being used and looked at it with a critical eye.

We have 13 weightlifting movements, nine gymnastics movements and eight monostructural movements. Actually, it could be 10 gymnastics and seven monostructural if I change the classification of the O-course. Right now, I have it listed as monostructural because of the sprint aspect of it, but it should really be in the gymnastics category.

At first glance, the list seems skewed toward weightlifting. But when I look into it, I think it's justified. Actually, I think the score between weightlifting and gymnastics is much more balanced. Here's why: For the odd-object event, I considered each implement one instance of weightlifting. If I treat the trio as one, it's 11 weightlifting movements. On that same note, I didn't consider each individual obstacle in the O-course an instance of gymnastics. I'm rationalizing this to myself, really, and the distribution of movements is fine. I have 11 weightlifting, 10 gymnastics and seven monostructural movements.

What I'm watching for—and avoiding—is a list that's skewed heavily in one direction. Something like 15 weightlifting movements, five gymnastics movements and four monostructural movements. That would be unbalanced programming in favor of the really strong athletes. Moving in the opposite direction would create a similar problem—five weightlifting movements, 14 gymnastics movements and four monostructrual movements. Those are extreme examples, but this is what I consider to ensure a fair test of fitness. I ensure all my checks and balances are in place when creating this test. It will be a true test of the Fittest on Earth.

Fitness is larger than the programming. The fittest will prevail regardless of what is programmed. For example, take Rich Froning and all his wins in the Open, at Regionals and at the Games. That's fitness. Mat Fraser has a chance to replicate aspects of Rich's performance, to always be on top regardless of the test. That's what we're looking for.

But it's possible to program the Games away from fitness and bias the programming toward the strongest of the really fit people, or maybe toward the really fit people who excel at body-weight movements. Loading of the weightlifting components is also another area to examine carefully, but not as part of this initial look.

By doing the exercise I just did, I see if the programming is skewing in one direction or the other. I do this with all my programming for events. I'm looking through the Games Finals now, but similar reviews are performed throughout every programming process, even when there are only a few events.

Another thing I looked at tonight was the number of elements per test—singles, couplets, triplets, fours, fives, etc. I count how many we have of each type. The breakdown looks like this: We have three single-modality tests—the bike, 1RM snatch and O-course. *(Again, the O-course could be defined a few different ways. For now, I'll consider it a single-element test.)*

We have six couplets, two triplets, one quad and one with five movements. So the programming is biased toward couplets—six of 13 events. Just under half. I'm OK with that because they're all very different in terms of movements, formats, time domains, etc. Most importantly, couplets are in line with CrossFit's charter, which holds that basic tests and workouts are often most effective.

People often get really caught up in making challenging, crazy chippers that involve a lot of movements or a lot of components. But the efficacy of a simple couplet is at the heart of CrossFit.

When looking at the couplets, I also list their type: MM, WG, WM, WG, WM, WG. Three of the six are WG, which is probably the most common and effective of the couplets in CrossFit. Weightlifting and gymnastics. Two others are weightlifting and monostructural, and one is monostructural and monostructural. It might have been nice to see a GG or a GM, but I feel comfortable with this distribution.

We have two triplets, and both are WGM—a classic expression. One triplet features running with cleans and burpees over hay walls. The interval test features rope climbs, overhead squats and SkiErgs.

Finally, we have the four-element odd-object event and the five-element chipper. The four-element test with the handstand walking is a very cool event that's not really *"traditional CrossFit,"* but it will be exciting. The five-element event is classic CrossFit—a high-rep chipper. Both of these events were created late in the game, and the five-movement chipper actually started as a three-modality test. But when analyzing everything throughout the process, I recognized a majority of couplets and triplets about a month ago. I was then able to make some adjustments that I think improved the tests.

A couple of cool notes about the four- and five-element tests: One is WWWG and the other is GGGWM. So both are biased in structure toward either weightlifting or gymnastics. But in actuality the tests are very well balanced internally by the interaction of their individual elements.

If you were paying attention earlier, I considered the WWWG event WG when balancing weightlifting and gymnastics movements, but in this subsequent analysis it makes more sense to consider it WWWG.

That said, maybe I should just consider the overall balance 13-10-7 weightlifting-gymnastics-monstructural. But it's in a place where I'm comfortable, and I don't view it as unbalanced at all because of what's happening in a lot of the tests.

Tomorrow, I'll dive into time domains, types of weightlifting movements and event format.

*Saturday, July 15, 11:38 a.m.*

I was thinking about how nice it's been without testing for the past couple of days. The last time we tested, I really wasn't feeling it. So two days at home without testing was a nice break. Tomorrow we're back at it. Julian will test the final event with the actual parallettes we'll use in Madison. I had Bill overnight a set to me. They're taller than the parallettes we were using and will create deeper handstand push-ups. After that, a majority of the testing will involve Team stuff. Paradiso CrossFit is coming down to help with that.

Speaking of Team events, as I was driving into Yarrow I had an idea for one of the Team tests I'm currently unhappy with: the run with the Worm and the burpee over the hay bales. We tested it for 5 rounds, and it was good, but it didn't affect the team as I was hoping it would. The more I think about it, I really don't like that one. When we were flying to Scotts Valley a few days ago, I told Stephane I didn't like it, and he suggested we make them carry a litter. I told him the litter wasn't really hard when we did it last year. It was just annoying. We agreed on that.

But as I was driving in, I wasn't really thinking about that event, but this idea hit me: Why don't I have three people run the course with the litter? That would be much harder than having four or five people carry it. While that happens, the other three athletes could do burpees over the hay bales. Conceptually, I like this. I'll just need to play with the reps and the distances to make sure the burpee people will be done or close to done when the athletes return with the litter. Those movements work well together, too. I just need to sketch out some ideas and see how it could work. I admit it would be hard to follow as a fan, but I think it's a much better test. I like this one. I'll work on that in a bit, but first I want to continue the analysis of Individual events.

I have 13 loaded elements in the Games, and I then broke them up into four categories: barbell, dumbbell, kettlebell and odd.

In the odd category, I have five movements: the Banger (*I consider it weightlifting because it involves controlling and managing an external load)*, the yoke, the farmers carry, the sled pull and the med-ball clean.

In the kettlebell category we have two movements: kettlebell deadlift and kettlebell overhead walking lunge.

In the dumbbell category we have one: the push press. This will be a welcome surprise for athletes who saw many dumbbells in the Open and at Regionals.

That's eight total non-barbell movements.

On the barbell side, we have five: the squat snatch *(light)*, the squat snatch *(heavy)*, the clean *(power or squat)*, the thruster and the OHS.

Now I take a look at what's heavy and what's light. I have seven classified as heavy and six classified as light. That's important so the programming is not just all heavy events and heavy tests. Now understand that when I say "*heavy*" and "*light*," some might actually fall into a "*medium*" category, and what's light for Games athletes is not light for 99 percent of the CrossFit world. But I have to look at what they are capable of, not what we are capable of.

The squat snatch on Day 1 is light. The 1RM is obviously heavy. The clean event can be considered light to heavy, but I just classified it as heavy. The thruster is light. The overhead squat is also light. The push press I categorized as heavy, but really it's medium or possibly even light. The Banger is light. The yoke, farmers carry and pull are all heavy. The med ball on the run event also gets a light ranking. It's very light by design, and I want them to rip through and just move on that event. The kettlebell deadlift also gets a heavy ranking, and the overhead lunge in that final gets a light designation.

That distribution of light to heavy loading in the programming looks fair to me.

Two things that stand out: There is a lot of squatting, and they do squat snatches two days in a row. At first glance, I'm not a fan of back-to-back days with squat snatches. But I'm fine with it because each instance is a very different expression of the movement. One version is light—again, light for them, not us. The other version is on the opposite end of the spectrum: a 1-rep max.

As for the squatting, we have high reps on Thursday and low reps but heavy weight on Friday. On Saturday we have the sprint clean ladder, in which athletes can use power cleans until they need to go to a squat, but that test has very few reps in total. Later that day, they have high-rep squats courtesy of the thrusters in the 17.5++ variation. On Sunday, they have high-rep overhead squats in the interval test.

So on Day 1, they squat, but the squats are very limited on Day 2. I say "limited" because the OHS portion of the heavy snatch is not the limiting factor in that movement. Day 3 and the final day also have high-rep squatting. That's fine. For athletes in the normal CrossFit world, that would be too much, but this programming is for the Fittest on Earth.

Let's take a look at the pulling. We have a light pull on Day 1 with the squat snatch, a heavy pull on Day 2 with the 1RM squat snatch, and the sled pull on Day 3. The sled work is a "true pull," but when I talk about pulling here, I'm generally talking about taking things from the ground. Later on Day 3, we have the clean ladder, which is a lot of pulling (it's paired with a lot of gymnastics pulling through bar muscle-ups). On Day 4, we have light pulling with the med-ball clean and then heavy pulling with the kettlebell deadlift.

In terms of pushing, we have the thruster and the push press.

Remember, at this stage we are only looking at the weightlifting movements. In total, I have five squats, six pulls and two pushes. In some instances, elements are found in the same movement. For example, the thruster has both a squat and a push.

I didn't include some of the odd objects in these categories.

In terms of gymnastics movements, we have pulling in Thursday's ring muscle-ups and Friday's pull-ups. The muscle-up also has a little push at the top, but I'm not going to count that. The GHD provides a great hip-closing movement at high reps, and this is the first time we have tested athletes on the GHD this season. We didn't use the movement at Regionals. The pistol provides a squatting gymnastics movement. On Saturday, we have the handstand walk, which can be considered a pushing element. Later in the same day, we have the bar muscle-up, which is another type of pull. On

Sunday we have the burpee, which is just annoying. The rope climb is a nice long pull, and the handstand push-ups in the final are obviously pushing.

So Day 1: pull. Day 2: pull, close hip, squat. Day 3: push, pull. Day 4: burpee, pull, push.

I would have liked to have seen one more closing of the hip—like toes-to-bars—but I'm not going to force it into the programming at this stage. I originally had hip closing in the chipper, but it's cleaner without.

Now I can take a look at all the events and see what's going on as a whole. Again, this process of evaluation is continually happening as I program. At this stage, I'm reviewing everything together.

Event 1, Run Swim Run: straightforward. Three metabolic elements.

Event 2, the bike: straightforward, too. It's gassy and leg intensive, but mostly it's about gas and grit.

Event 3, longer Amanda: pulling and pushing on the rings, and pulling on the barbell combined with light squatting.

Event 4, O-course: This can be considered a lot of pulling, but it will not be demanding pulling because it will be so fast.

Event 5, chipper: We have pull (pull-up), hip close (GHD), squat (pistol), pull (row) and push (dumbbell push press). I have two instances of pulling in the same event, but they are very different in terms of plane of action, and they're separated by other functions that all tie it together.

Event 6, the 1RM squat snatch. Big pull, big squat.

Event 7, the Banger and Assault bike: metabolic nightmare combined with another nightmare.

Event 8, strongman: some odd objects with some handstand walks.

Event 9, clean ladder: big pull with big pull. The clean is loaded and originates on the ground. In the muscle-up, the athlete starts in the hang and moves to support on top of a bar. So both pulls have a bar. In one, the athlete takes the bar from below and brings it to the shoulders. In the other, the bar is fixed and the athlete moves from below to above. In the clean, they pull a heavy weight. In the muscle-up, they pull their body weight. Both movements require the full body, as well as sound technique for efficient performance. Even though it's pull and pull, it's a beautiful pairing. Simple and effective.

Event 10, 17.5++: thrusters and double-unders—just gassing them. The movement functions here are fine paired together.

Event 11, med-ball burpee and run: a light pull followed by a full-body movement over the hay bale, then short-distance running, at least compared to the running distance on Day 1.

Event 12, the intervals: a big pull on the rope climb, plus closing of the hip and downward pulling on the SkiErg. Nice to see another good test of closing of the hip. And then squatty with OHS.

Event 13, the final: pushing with the kipping handstand push-ups on parallettes, combined with heavy, short pulls via deadlifts. And then lunges while stabilizing weight overhead.

*4:04 p.m.*
I just got back to Yarrow for the second analyzing session of the day. I want to dive into the format and setup of the events.

We have three single-modality tests: the 1RM snatch, the bike and the O-course. That's a nice distribution: weightlifting, monostructural, gymnastics. An argument could be made that the O-course features multiple gymnastics elements, but I'm going to consider it a single element. The snatch is a nice heavy test, the bike is a longer-distance test, and the O-course is a sprint event. I'll analyze time domains later.

We have six couplets, and each has a very different look.

Run Swim Run (MM) is a race that starts with one movement, goes to another and returns to the first movement. It could be considered a *"couplet chipper"* in format.

The longer Amanda (GW) is a traditional couplet that pairs a gymnastics movement with a barbell movement. The load is fixed, and the reps decrease.

The bike/Banger couplet (MW) is a sprint chipper with two elements.

The squat-clean/bar-muscle-up test (WG) is a couplet with fixed rounds and fixed reps but increasing loads. This is our only traditional CrossFit test that has ascending weight this year.

17.5++ (WM) is a very traditional couplet with fixed reps and rounds.

Finally, the handstand-push-up/kettlebell-deadlift couplet features fixed rounds and ascending reps. It's the only event with ascending reps.

These couplets are all very different in format but still classic CrossFit for the most part. They'll give athletes and fans plenty to geek out over.

The two triplets are both MGW—a classic setup—but they're very different in layout.

The run/clean/burpee triplet features fixed rounds and reps. The other, the interval test, also features fixed reps, but the format is unique. I'm very excited about this one. We've spent a ton of time tweaking it to get it right. This one is going to be amazing, and it will be the first true interval event we do at the Games.

For the four- and five-modality tests, each has a unique look.

The four-modality event is unique, and I don't know how to categorize it. Athletes move objects across the field and perform handstand walks when they aren't carrying something. It will make for a great show in Madison.

The five-modality test is a classic high-rep chipper (GGGMW). It starts off with a lot of high-rep body-weight stuff and ends with some big-kid stuff. This one will be fun to watch, too.

I'll analyze the timing later. I did one analysis a few weeks ago, and everything is where it needs to be for me to be content. But I'll dive into it probably tomorrow or Monday. I have to step away to check the Team events I'm testing tomorrow. I need to get my head around what we're going to have them do. The events are kinda complicated, and I'm getting tired, so I don't really feel like typing them out right now.

I also put some thought into the event with the litter run and the burpees. I'll probably need to test that in Madison, but I might be able to get it done here. Maybe next weekend. Actually, that's what I should do. That way we are more prepared. I'll text Bill now and tell him we need a litter. I don't have one anymore. Last year, I took it up to the Games and gave it back to Bill and the Rogue crew. I didn't think I would need it this year, but I guess I should have held onto it. I also recently returned the three bales of hay. I guess I might need to buy more so I can create the wall for the team. I'm thinking something like run the litter 200 or 300 meters with three people—two carrying it and one on it. The other three athletes are doing a fixed number of burpees during that time. Oh yeah—all of this with body armor, too. So the litter really makes sense, and it's a perfect place for body armor. The big thing to test is the timing. I want the burpee reps to take roughly the same time it takes the trio to run the litter around a fixed course.

I also have Julian coming early tomorrow to test the final with the deep parallettes. I'm having him come early so the team won't see that go down.

This evening, Robert Guerrero is fighting, and I'm excited. Robert is a friend, and I organized training for him through CrossFit. About four or five fights ago, he trained with Brian Chontosh and won the fight. After that, he backed off CrossFit for the last three fights, and he lost two of them. About six months ago, he hit me up and said he's ready to seriously get back into CrossFit. I said he needed to get into it in the offseason, out of camp, and that's what he did. He started training a lot months before he had a fight scheduled, so he entered his fight camp in great shape.

He's going into the fight tonight against an undefeated, hungry, younger fighter. For Robert, it's basically win or think about hanging up the gloves. I really hope his CrossFit training over the last six months will trump his age. I hope CrossFit can extend his career. We'll find out shortly.

*Sunday, July 16, 4:36 p.m.*
Today was a very long day of testing, and it was very good. I'll get to that. First, I want to talk about the fight last night.

Robert lost, and that was disappointing. He came in looking great and started the first round with an aggressive pace. He was pushing forward and landing some great shots. His opponent looked timid and wasn't really throwing anything. One of the commentators said his opponent takes a round or two to warm up.

Sure enough, he was warmed up in Round 2. They were fighting on the inside and he hit Robert with a massive uppercut. The fight changed at that moment. Robert went down. He got up and continued to press in, but he ended up getting knocked down two more times in that round. I'm really surprised the referee didn't stop it after the third knockdown. In Round 3, Robert came out hot, rushed to the center of the ring to brawl and started landing some great blows. But they got in tight, and that's where this guy was doing all his damage with uppercuts and power punches. Robert went down again. And then a moment later he went down a second time. After that, the ref stopped the fight.

It was hard to watch. I've watched Robert fight a number of times, and I've never seen him get knocked down that much. This morning, I texted Greg Amundson and asked him if they had talked about retiring last night. He said yes, that had come up. I think that's the best decision for Robert at this stage in his career. He's had a great career, he has a great family, and he has a great future. He should take it easy and step away from the punishment.

This morning, I showed up to Yarrow at 7:30. I did the CrossFit.com WOD before Julian arrived. It was a good one, and it kicked my ass. It was a chipper with 50 reps of five movements. It was similar to something we did the other day. Both workouts ended with 50 burpees. I compared my burpee time to that of two days ago, and today's set was about 45 seconds faster. I'm happy about that.

Once Julian showed up, we played some knockout games, and then I told him to warm up for the final—5-8-13 reps of parallette handstand push-ups and kettlebell deadlifts. This time we have the parallettes we'll use at the Games. They're about 3 or 4 inches higher than the ones we've been testing with. The depth of the HSPU is significant. I told Julian I just wanted him to test the first section, not the lunge part. I didn't need to see that again. I know it works well.

5-8-13 REPS OF:

PARALLETTE HANDSTAND PUSH-UPS

KETTLEBELL DEADLIFTS (200 LB.)

The first set of handstand push-ups took 17 seconds. Julian came off the wall once, not because of fatigue but because he lost his balance. He finished the first 5 deadlifts at 33 seconds.

He had to break the 8 HSPU into 2 sets of 4, and he was done with the deadlifts at 1:30.

The set of 13 handstand push-ups was a game changer. It was drastically different from his set on the lower parallettes in previous testing. He started with a set of 3, then did a set of 5, which took him to 2:11. From that point on it was singles all the way to 13, and Julian missed a couple, too. Julian struggled on that last set, and he considers handstand push-ups a strength. He was surprised, as were we.

His total time was 4:07. The last time he tested this event, he finished the couplet at 2:37, and his total time was 4:11. Today it was 4:07 without the lunges.

After seeing the difficulty of the set of 13 parallette HSPU, I think the test is perfect this way. It's very cool to see the first 2 rounds go by fast before the third changes the game. I'll probably have a girl test it soon, and the 3-5-8 rep scheme is probably perfect for them. I like the added challenge of the depth.

After Julian was done, the Paradiso CrossFit team rolled in from Venice, California. They made the Games a few years back, and this year they were a spot or two away from qualifying again.

We started with a Team Worm event—the one I'm planning on having the teams do on Saturday.

IN PAIRS, 30 PULL-UPS EACH, 25 TOES-TO-BARS EACH, 15/12 CALORIES EACH ON THE SKIERG

12 WORM CLEANS AS A TEAM

IN PAIRS, 30 PULL-UPS EACH, 25 TOES-TO-BARS EACH, 15/12 CALORIES EACH ON THE SKIERG

12 WORM CLEANS AS A TEAM

IN PAIRS, 30 PULL-UPS EACH, 25 TOES-TO-BARS EACH, 15/12 CALORIES EACH ON THE SKIERG

12 WORM CLEANS AS A TEAM

EACH ROUND, PAIRS COMPLETE A DIFFERENT EXERCISE

On go, six athletes will head out to the four-person rig. Two will do 30 pull-ups, two will do 25 toes-to-bars and the other two will do 15/12 calories on the SkiErg. The reps do not have to be synchronized. The athletes just need to get the work done. I hope I've programmed the reps so they all finish within a few seconds of each other. When they're done with everything, they go to the Worm for 12 cleans. They'll do 3 rounds of that. Each time they come back to the rig, the pairs will do a different movement. At the end, each teammate will have done 30 pull-ups, 25 toes-to-bars and 15 or 12 calories on the SkiErg. Everyone is pretty much working at the same time, which is cool. There's no room to rest.

After we started the clock, they ran to their positions and finished the first round's individual work in 54 seconds. A few finished sooner than the others, but not by much. At the Worm—the heavy one—they were confused about where to place each athlete. They finished 12 cleans at 2:03.

At this point, they all returned to the rig and the SkiErgs and rotated to a different position. In this round, the first athlete finished at 2:49 and the last at 3:08—about 20 seconds' difference in rest from first to last. Lauren Gravatt was the first to finish. She's the sister of longtime CrossFit affiliate owner Jordan Gravatt, who is a good friend of mine. Generally speaking, she was the anchor, leader and star of the team all day.

The second set of cleans was much harder for them. They finished at 4:40, about 1:30 after starting the set. You could really see the cleans were becoming difficult and the extra weight was taking its toll.

On the third and final set of individual work, Lauren was again the first to finish. Her last station was toes-to-bars, and she finished at 5:35. Everyone else finished about 10-15 seconds after her, except for the other guy on toes-to-bars. He was the slow one, and the team left that section at 6:08. They logged their first clean at 6:17 and started fighting for reps. They missed the ninth rep because the Worm was just devastating them. They also missed on Rep 11. They ended up finishing with a total time of 7:50.

They were blasted, and I liked the way it looked. Later, when I sat down to take a look at this test in relation to the other events and the schedule, I decided to make some changes. I want to increase the work at each station, as well as the reps on the Worm. I think we'll do something like this: 40 pull-ups, 30 toes-to-bars and 18/13 calories on the SkiErg. Then we'll have them do a larger number of Worm cleans, with a descending pattern of 17-15-12. I figure this should take slightly longer, maybe 8-11 minutes. This event has an 11-minute cap, so the change should be fine for the Games teams.

I want to increase the reps because that set of pull-ups is basically the only set of pull-ups they'll do at the Games, and 30 sounds low. Forty is low.

But 40 sounds better to me than 30. As for the increase in Worm cleans, well, this is the Games and they should come prepared.

I let the team recover for about 10-15 minutes, and then we hit another one. Julian had to sub in because one of the team members was wrecked and couldn't really do another event right away. As of right now, this would be the final event for the teams, and it features the Worm.

I had them do 2 rounds of the following: They all pick up a light Worm, then hold in place while two people leave. Those two go to a rope and a wall. One person does 15 handstand push-ups while the other does 2 rope climbs. Once they finish, they switch and finish the reps. Then they both head back to the Worm, and two other athletes head to the rope and wall. So every athlete does 2 rope climbs and 15 handstand push-ups, and four people hold the Worm while the others work. Then they all go to the large Worm and do a clean complex with 10 reps. They clean the Worm to the shoulders, squat it, drop it, step over and repeat on the other side. The team will do 2 rounds of all this.

2 ROUNDS OF:

WHILE TEAM HOLDS WORM, PAIRS EACH PERFORM 2 ROPE CLIMBS AND 15 HSPU

10 WORM COMPLEXES*

*WORM COMPLEX = 1 CLEAN, 1 SQUAT, DROP, STEP OVER

On the first round, they picked up the light Worm and two athletes left to work. Each finished the rope climbs/handstand push-ups in 35 seconds. Then they switched and finished the second part of their work at 1:05. They ran back to the Worm and switched out with two other athletes, who were able to finish all their work at 2:14. The third pair finished at 3:17. The teammates ran to the big Worm and started the clean complex. They finished 5 reps in about 40 seconds, and they had completed 10 by 4:48.

They finished the second round with the light Worm at 8:16. As they were setting up on the heavy Worm, I told them to do 2 squats for every clean. This time the first 5 took 50 seconds and the second 5 took about a minute. Their total time to finish was 10:54.

I liked it better with the second squat. I decided to add that on the fly to make the event more challenging without changing it too much. I haven't decided what I'm going to do with this one, but I am going to change it. I might increase the last section to 20 reps so they really have to fight. I don't know yet. I have to play with this one some more, write out some options, etc. I'll probably finalize it tomorrow.

After that, we took a break and I honestly thought they were done. Lauren pushed them and asked me, *"What else do you have?"* I didn't want them to feel like they were leaving empty handed, so I had them test the pairs relay event.

AS PAIRS COMPLETE:

16-20-24 SYNCHRO BAR MUSCLE-UPS (IN SETS OF 4)

50 GHD SIT-UPS

THEN, 2 ROUNDS OF:

16/12 CALORIES ON THE ASSAULT BIKE

10-12-14 REPS OF PARTNER DEADLIFTS

I told them they could use any pairings they wanted on the first part, but on the second it had to be mixed pairs. That's because one side of the deadlift bar is loaded up with five 45s and the other side is loaded up with five 55s.

They chose to use mixed pairs for the first part. Right away, one of the females struggled on the muscle-ups. *"Great, this is going to take them forever, and it won't give me a good time to analyze,"* I thought. Every rep she did looked very labored, as if she were going to miss. Surprisingly, she got through the first 3 sets of 4 without too much issue. On the last set, she missed a few, but they finished that section in 2:14. Not too bad, and not as bad as I thought it would be when I saw her start. They finished 50 GHDs at 4:23.

Pair 2 was much faster even though they had 4 additional bar muscle-ups. They finished everything at 8:15, for a time of about 3:52 for their first couplet—about 30 seconds faster than the first pair.

The final pair finished at 13:01. The female struggled with the 24 bar muscle-ups. She's actually really good at them, but when Julian Alcaraz is your partner, you're pushed to a point where you start missing. Honestly, I don't think Julian was pushing her. He was just keeping the pace and she couldn't hold it.

In the second couplet, the deadlift is really heavy. Everyone who has tested this event has said that. That's why the reps are low. The first pair finished at 16:37, giving them a time of 3:36. They struggled on the deadlift, and Round 2 was particularly hard for them. The second pair finished at 20:14 after cruising through the deadlifts, even though they did 24 total. Their time was about 3:37 for this couplet. The final pair finished the event at 24:30, with a time of about 4:15 for the couplet with 14 deadlifts. The second set of 14 really did them in, and they broke it multiple times.

I have the cap at 21 minutes, and they were about 3:30 over it. I told Stephane that I want to drop the reps on the deadlifts but still keep it hard. He suggested we use the same total number of reps as we're using for bar muscle-ups. At first I didn't understand. He explained: The first pair does 16 bar muscle-ups, so make the first deadlift sets 8 and 8—16 total. The second pair does 20 bar muscle-ups, so make the second pair's deadlifts 10 and 10. The third pair would do 12 and 12. Great idea. I liked that a lot. If I lower the reps a little, it will speed things up, and as an added benefit it will link the events numerically.

I eventually played with the cals on the Assault bike and decided on trying 15/10. That equals 25. Multiply 25 by 2 rounds and you get 50, the number of GHD sit-ups. Perfect. This one is settled. I love it. I just hope teams can do it all under 21 minutes. But I'm not worried about it. I analyzed it based off expected split times for fast teams, and I get right around 19:30-20:00. Under the cap by 1 minute.

And I don't care if some teams can't finish before the cap. They won't be the teams that matter.

*Monday, July 17, 12:58 p.m.*
I came into Yarrow about an hour ago. I've been looking at the Team events and the schedule. I'm pretty happy with everything but Sunday. I don't like the final event we tested or where it's currently at. I want to do something else, something similar in concept—but better. I also still don't like the Sunday-morning run event. I need to play with that one a little, take my pencil to paper and really write it out, see what's happening.

I'm really happy we didn't have any testing today. It's nice that it's finally winding down. I might test one or two things before I leave for Madison in about a week, and I'll have plenty to test out there.

I'm really happy to be at this place with the Games right now. I'm feeling good about everything, where we're at and how the planning is going. I feel good personally. Not stressed. Having almost two full weeks at home before traveling for the Games has been good for my head. I'm trying to zip everything up to be well rested by the time I head out there.

Last night, I announced the obstacle-course event with a picture from the 2012 O-course. I wanted to remind people that we did an obstacle-course event before obstacle-course races were cool or even a thing. The one we do here will be very unique to us, not like what the others are doing. It will be short and fast, like Pendleton was, and it will have a military feel and look to it, not like the current obstacle-course events out there.

*2:02 p.m.*

I haven't made much progress on the Team stuff. I have some ideas, but nothing is sticking. I think maybe I need to step away today and come back tomorrow. Or I just wait until we get there. Get some inspiration from being on scene. That usually happens. I get very creative at the event on the actual competition floors.

But it would be good to have everything buttoned up before we get there. It would be a CrossFit Games first for sure if I were able to pull that off.

But today I step away.

*Tuesday, July 18, 6:39 p.m.*

This morning I had a meeting with Adrian and Stephane, and at the last minute we added Mike Giardina. Adrian is the head judge for the Individual events, and Mike is the assistant head judge. In years past, Adrian's assistants have been Joe Alexander and E.C. Synkowski. This year, Mike is taking that role. He lives near me in Carlsbad, so it was easy to add him to the meeting.

The meeting allowed us to go over all the Individual events and answer any questions Boz might have. He knew them all from the meeting we had in Madison a few weeks ago, but we've made a ton of little changes and tweaks since then, so it was good to get him up to speed on what's current. We started on Day 1 and went through every Individual event in order. We looked at the floors and the schedule for each. It was a very good meeting. It lasted a little over two hours, and we got a ton done. Typically, this type of meeting would happen first thing when we get to the Games venue. It's a huge plus to knock it out now.

We discussed details of the cyclocross race, including how we're going to score it and how we're going to run the time trial day on Wednesday. We didn't make any decisions on scoring, just discussed pros and cons. I told Boz we'd have a discussion in Madison with Justin and Dave Eubanks, our scoring lead. Thinking this through, maybe we set up a call with this team to discuss this week or next so we don't have to figure it out in Madison.

We also discussed the pros and cons of letting the athletes practice on the O-course. Justin wants to let them practice. He even suggested using a time trial to seed them. I'm less into the time trial. I don't like that idea. But I'm considering the argument to let them practice. I could go either way at this point. I want to give it more thought.

We also made a list of all the things that need to be tested in Madison, and the list is longer than I thought. It includes the cyclocross course, the O-course—we obviously can't test those here. We also have to test the Banger event—especially the female version. I didn't have a female setup here, so I was only able to test the male version. We need to test the odd-object/handstand-walk event because we don't know how the sled will move on the turf. And we might need to test the final because I don't have access to enough good women here to get a lot of runs through it. I have Lindsey Valenzuela coming tomorrow to run through it, but I want a few more women to go through. I'll probably use all the Demo Team ladies. I want to see how the really deep parallettes affect them.

Before Stephane took Adrian to the airport, we played a game of knockout. I won the first round, then took dead last in the next 2 rounds. Adrian took the overall victory. Damn it. I love beating Adrian. I hardly ever beat him in CrossFit events anymore. There was a time when I would, but not these days, so when we play knockout I put him in my crosshairs.

I'm now going to take a look at the time domains of all the Individual events. I labeled them out on a timeline and listed what I think will be fast times or average fast times for each. It helps a lot to see all the time domains—and I noticed something that I'm going to change after this review.

Let's start with the longer events and work backward. Run Swim Run will be the longest event, anywhere from 27 to 28 minutes for the fastest to 40-45 for the slowest. I considered increasing the run distances to make it a little longer, but I'm fine with this window for the longest event this year. The test, whether I extend it or not, will do what we need it to do.

The next longest test is the cyclocross event. It's going to be 3 laps around the track, and it should take them 25-30 minutes. We'll test once we get there. Both of those long events are on Thursday, so we get them out of the way right away but also tax the athletes with these long efforts right out of the gate.

Those two events are basically not true CrossFit events in my sense of "*true*." They are part of the Games and part of the overall plan to test the athletes' overall fitness and skill. But if you just took those two tests in isolation, they're not pure CrossFit. The longest pure CrossFit event is the run/clean/burpee test with the hay bales. I have that one timed at about 18-20 minutes for the fastest. I'm excited about it, and its placement on Sunday means athletes will have to dig deep to go fast.

Next, based off my picture graph, I kinda have a gap between that event and the next timelines, which are in the range of 10-12 minutes. In that range, I basically have four events. I have the chipper Paul finished in 11-something. I have Amanda with the extra rounds, which Connor finished in 11-something. The interval test is basically 9 minutes of work if you cap, but Julian did it in 8:11. And 17.5++ is 9:30-11:00.

Seeing this cluster of events around 9-11 minutes caused me to confirm a change I had mentioned to Boz earlier today: adding more reps to the pull-ups on the chipper. If Paul did it in 11-something, the top guys will go 10 and even under 10. So I'm going to increase the reps to target a finish in the range of 12-13 minutes. The event has a 14-minute cap, so it would be good to lengthen it. Now that I plan on making a change, I might take a look at all its reps and change them all. I'll put pen to paper tomorrow and see how I can make the numbers work.

In the range of 6-8 minutes, we have the muscle-up/clean event. I think that will take 6-8 minutes for most. We also have the odd-object/handstand-walk event, which will probably be 8-10 minutes.

For shorter events, we have the final, which should end up being 4-6 minutes for most—high 4 for the fastest.

The Banger event is even faster. It's going to take anywhere from 2:30 to 3:00, so that's a true sprint event. The O-course is going to be about 1-2 minutes. We'll confirm the time in Madison.

The fastest event will be the 1RM snatch. That powerful effort only takes a couple of seconds.

Overall, I'm happy with the variation in the time domains. I have a couple of concerns. I'm wondering if I'm going to hate not taking Run Swim Run closer to 40 minutes. I don't think I will, but I find myself asking the question. I already addressed my other concern by making the chipper a little longer to remove the cluster of events in that 10-minute zone.

At this stage, the analysis of the Individual events is almost done. That analysis highlighted one big change I need to make to the chipper, but other than that everything seems to be solid and the events play well off each other.

Another thing I need to do: name them. I'll start working on that tomorrow. Some will have simple names. For example, the obstacle course will be O-Course. The actual CrossFit events will get little names. Not sure on all of them yet.

I'm about 10 days away from leaving and still haven't figured out two Team events. Well, that's not true. I have them in place, and I have things we tested. But I'm not 100 percent happy with them. I need to refine them.

I'll do a similar analysis of the Team events, but it won't be as in depth and it won't have the same goals. For the Team events, I'm more worried about testing their ability to function together as a cohesive unit while performing functional movements executed at high intensity.

*Wednesday, July 19, 5:10 p.m.*
Fuck, I turn 40 tomorrow.

Today is my last day in my 30s. It's been a fun ride, my 30s. I can't imagine the next 10 years won't be anything but more of the same, or they'll be even more incredible. I view my 20s largely as defined by my time in the Navy, and CrossFit defined my 30s. There were some years of overlap, but that delineation is an easy way to look at my life.

This afternoon, Lindsey came by to test a couple of things for me. First, we had her test the 3-5-8 final with the deep Rogue parallettes. When we first had her play with them, she couldn't get out of the hole. That's how deep they are. I think they're 14 inches. We've used them before with female athletes at the 2015 Games, so Stephane checked video footage of that event, and we saw that we had put tiles down to reduce the depth. We recreated the tile setup and reduced the depth by 3 inches. For Lindsey, that was the difference between not being able to do any and being able to knock out reps.

After making sure the height was correct, we kicked off.

3-5-8 REPS OF:

PARALLETTE HANDSTAND PUSH-UPS

KETTLEBELL DEADLIFTS (124 LB.)

Lindsey finished the set of 3 handstand push-ups at 8 seconds and the deadlifts at 18 seconds.

On her second round, she decided to do 3 and 2 on the wall. She finished that set at 50 seconds. Her set of 5 deadlifts was unbroken and complete at 1:07.

She started the set of 8 with 2, and I could tell this round would not be easy. She went to some singles, and toward the end of the round she rested a bit more and was able to do a couple of sets of 2. The final handstand push-up was locked out at 3:15, meaning it took her 1 minute to do the first 2 rounds and then more than 2 minutes to finish the set of 8 HSPU. She knocked the deadlifts out to finish at 3:37.

I didn't have her do the final set of lunges. I don't really need that tested at this stage. I just want to see the timing of the first part. I'm mostly happy with the women's version, but as I was thinking about it, I wondered if we should just do 2 rounds—8 and 13 reps, like the last two rounds of the men's version. Instead of 5-8-13, maybe it's just 8-13. That would increase the difficulty of the deadlifts without creating a huge number of handstand push-ups. The deadlifts in the version Lindsey just tested are easy.

Or perhaps I could just use the men's deadlift scheme and reduce the number of handstand push-ups: 3-5-8 HSPU and 5-8-13 deadlifts. Hmm, that might slow it down too much. Really, the deadlift is easy. It's all handstand push-ups. But that's OK.

This gives me more to think about for the women's version. I like the idea of a different rep scheme. We're less than a few weeks away, but I'm still sweating the details of this stuff, as I should be.

After that test, we had Lindsey warm up for the muscle-up/clean event. I had her test this event with that twist: She's the first athlete who will do the bar muscle-ups in singles. Everyone who tested it was able to do all 4 reps in 1 set. But I now know we will have a rig with four bars in each lane, so the athletes can do a rep and then advance to the next bar.

## 4 BAR MUSCLE-UPS AS SINGLES

## 2 CLEANS (145, 160, 175, 190, 205, 215, 225, 235 LB.)

We had set the workout up so she had a different bar for each muscle-up, and the first 4 singles took her 20 seconds. She commented on how annoying it was as she finished that set. I liked hearing that. That's the point. She finished her first 2 cleans at 33 seconds.

She finished the next 4 muscle-ups at 1:07, and then power-cleaned the second weight twice to finish at 1:23.

The next round's muscle-ups were complete at 1:57. She moved to the 175-lb. bar and again power-cleaned both reps, finishing at 2:18.

The fourth round of gymnastics was complete at 2:57, and she power-cleaned 190 twice to move back to the rig at 3:20.

Every rep on the barbell was a single. Even the early ones. Her pace on the muscle-ups was consistent—slow and deliberate.

Her fifth set of muscle-ups was finished at 3:58. For the 205 bar, Lindsey belted up and took a little more time setting up, but she still power-cleaned both reps as singles, finishing the second rep at 4:39. She ripped her belt off and threw it to the next bar.

I was impressed with the fact that she was still using power cleans. If we were working side by side on the same test with the same weight, she would be crushing me right now.

Her sixth set of bar muscle-ups was a tad slower. She needed a little more rest before each. She finished the last one at 5:23. On the 215 bar, she went to a squat clean for the first time, and she took more rest between reps. She finished her second clean at 6:24.

On her seventh set, she did something interesting: She cranked them out. She did a rep, dropped, moved over and quickly did another. She was much faster on the muscle-ups and moved to the barbell at 7:03. She looked ready for 225. She set up, pulled and then dropped under. It looked labored and slow, but she got it up. Lindsey took a good rest before coming back and going for the second. She got that rep at 8:30, unbelted.

She once again finished the bar muscle-ups quickly. At 9:03 she was to the 235-lb. bar. She chalked up, put her belt on again and gained her composure. She waited about a minute before making her first attempt. She got under it and fell straight backward, landing on her back. I asked her if she wanted to make another attempt and she said yes. She got under it, but she couldn't stand up, so we stopped. That was at the 11-minute mark, and this event has a cap of 10 minutes. She would have hit the cap around her first attempt at 235.

Of the three women who have tested it, Lindsey went the deepest. She's known for her strength, but some of the girls in the Games field are even stronger, so they should have no problem with the weight. I'm very happy with where this event is at.

Today Pat and Stephane let me know that the Team Series events are basically due now, so we'll have a look at those in the next few days or next week so I can sign off on them before I head to Madison. Pat made the events already, and I just have to give them a once over. Really, the process is a little more complicated than that. He drafts them out, and I look through them, edit them, make changes and then send them back as the final. Regardless of the process, I'm really annoyed that I have to get those done at this point.

I'm getting ready to go home to have my last meal in my 30s. I'll accompany that with the last drink of my 30s.

I'm old.

*Thursday, July 20, 8:28 p.m.*
I'm old.

I didn't do a lot at Yarrow. I took the day off from testing with athletes. I mostly read and did other CrossFit work. I'm currently reading *"The Iliad"* by Homer. Great book. I'm enjoying it more than I enjoyed *"The Odyssey."* I need to reread *"Odyssey"*—but a different translation. This is something James Hobart recommended I do. The translation I read was by Robert Fagles.

I think I made progress with the Team event I was stuck on. Today while showering, I had an idea, and I've spent some time thinking it through. The event we tested had 2 rounds of rope climbs, handstand push-ups and

Worm cleans. I'm thinking of having them do 3 rounds of just rope climbs and handstand push-ups, then a large set of Worm cleans. It will be like two events in one. In the first round, every athlete does 1 rope climb and 10 HSPU, with two athletes working while four hold a light Worm. Once everyone is done, they cycle through again, this time doing 2 rope climbs and 15 HSPU. On Round 3, they'll do 3 rope climbs and 20 HSPU. Once all that is done—without giving it too much thought, I think it will take 5-7 minutes—they do 30 to 40 reps of the Worm complex. I like this version much more. It makes for a good race at the end if teams are evenly matched going into that part. It also gives a different look to the traditional Worm events. As they were written, they all looked similar.

Tomorrow Julian is coming over, and we're going to have him test the new version of the chipper. After a handful of edits, my first version was 80 pull-ups, 60 GHD sit-ups, 50 pistols, 40 calories and 20 push presses. The new, longer version will be 100 pull-ups, 80 GHDs, 60 pistols, 40 calories and 20 push presses. I think I'll like this version a lot.

*Friday, July 21, 6:24 a.m.*

I had a nightmare last night that woke me up at 4 in the morning. I was with all the Individual athletes on the Friday of the Games, and we were getting ready to do the Banger event. But I realized we had completely forgotten to do an event.

I ran to Justin and said, *"Hey, what's that event? I forgot what it was."* He had forgotten, too, but after some deliberation we remembered it had toes-to-bars and running. I was like, *"Fuck. Another event also has toes-to-bars, so we to need to change it."*

I started trying to figure out a new event on the spot as all the athletes stood around wondering what was going on.

*1:51 p.m.*

Today at 10 a.m., Julian met us to test the chipper with the additional reps. We warmed up a little and played basketball, of course. Then he attacked it.

100 PULL-UPS

80 GHD SIT-UPS

60 PISTOLS

40 CALORIES ON THE ROWER

20 DUMBBELL PUSH PRESSES (100 LB., SWITCHING ARMS EVERY 5 REPS)

Julian was much slower on the pull-ups than I expected. I think he tore his hand early on, and he finished at 3:36. Consider that Paul and Kelley did their sets of 80 in about 1:30-1:40. A set of 100 is a different beast, though, and it has to be attacked in a different way. I can see how athletes view 80 as more of a sprint, while 100 makes them more conservative. Let's say Paul and Kelley had to do a set of 100 each. They did 80 in 1:30, so it's safe to assume that they could have done 100 in 2:00-2:30. That's important to remember when I consider the overall time for this test. Their total projected time for 100 pull-ups was about 1 minute faster than Julian's actual time. He broke the set up a lot. He stopped at 15 and then did small sets all the way up. Paul and Kelley had opened with sets of 45 and 50, respectively, then finished 80 with 2 additional sets.

The 80 GHD sit-ups took Julian about 4:15. He took a couple of breaks, but they were short. I imagine this section will be about 3:45-4:00, but not much faster. GHDs just eat up time, and they're consistent in cycle speed for the most part. His total time was 8:01 at that point.

He completed his first 20 pistols in about 50 seconds, and his next 20 took the same amount of time. He sped up for his last set of 20 and finished them in about 44 seconds, bringing his total time to 10:24.

Julian started rowing at 10:44, and it took him past 11:30—essentially when Paul had finished the shorter version. He eventually finished rowing at 13:05.

He ripped the first set of 10 push presses in 20 seconds and put the dumbbell down. Then he did a set of 5. He added an additional set of 5 to finish the entire test in 14:20.

This rep scheme put the test in a better time domain. I still think it will end up being about 12:30-13:00, but that's better than 10-11 minutes. I have a cluster of other tests in that realm.

There are going to be three sticking points in this one. The pull-ups will slow some athletes down a lot, and the GHDs will work over those who didn't prepare properly. Of course, the 100-lb. dumbbell (*70 for the women*) will eat some people up. We talked about it briefly and Josh Bridges was mentioned, but I think he'll be fine on the dumbbell. Cody Anderson, on the other hand—I think he'll struggle with it. Ryan Elrod might struggle with it, too.

Actually, we just notified Ryan today that he will be banned from competing in the Games for two years for failing a drug test. We banned two other athletes, one from a team in San Diego and one from a team in the Northwest. They will both get two-year suspensions, and their teams won't be allowed to compete.

After getting the news from us, Ryan emailed us. He was very angry and emotional, and I can understand why. It must be heartbreaking. Then he took to Instagram to defend himself and announce the decision to his followers. Basically, he was taking a fertility drug—and something in that is banned. That's why he failed the test. Justin put out a statement that said athletes have to be accountable for what they put in their bodies. Even if something was prescribed or taken with the best intentions in the world, we can't tolerate it if it goes against our testing protocol.

I've been at Yarrow for a few hours today in addition to the testing. Earlier, Stephane had mentioned that I have very little time for the male-female transition on 17.5++. The issue here is that we are doing it with 10 bars—10 bars across 10 lanes, 100 bars on the floor. I had 5 minutes to make the transition happen, and it could be done in 5. But to make everyone happy—the logistics teams, the gear teams, the people in charge of the transitions—I added an additional 5. So now that transition is 10 minutes. Ten bars per minute—easy day. Oh, and they have 2 minutes from the last heat and 2 minutes from the next heat built in, so it's really 14 minutes for the transition. Again, plenty of time.

I went through the schedule again in detail and made some slight adjustments, reducing break times and changing some small things like that. Nothing too major.

No testing tomorrow. I'll come in and dive into some Team stuff again. I'm testing Team workouts on Sunday with Paradiso. Hopefully that will be the last testing session before I leave on Friday, seven days from now.

*Sunday, July 23, 8:04 p.m.*
Testing with the team went well this morning. They came with a different cast of men, and two of the women were the same. The third woman they brought was a tall, built girl I later found out was a national-champion swimmer at Arizona.

We had them do all of Sunday's events, which, at this point, were still works in progress. The run/burpee event was one of the first I had tested, but after thinking about it, I really didn't like how it played out. After a lot of sketching and modeling, and some discussions with Stephane, I decided to include the litter. The inclusion of the litter in last year's Games was anticlimactic in my mind. It was more of a nuisance than a real challenge. That's because we had one athlete on it and four carrying, but the sixth athlete didn't have to do anything. This year, I'm going to have two athletes carrying a third. The litter will move around a course while the other three are doing burpees over hay bales.

In the first version I created, they all ran with the Worm and they all did burpees at the same time. But the burpees were kinda slow, and the testing athletes recovered in that section. In this version, with three people doing burpees, the intensity will stay high.

Before deciding on the reps for the burpees, I had a team run around the building. The distance was 250 meters, and it took them about 1:45. Then I asked the other trio to do 15 burpees over the hay. That took about 1:45, but they did something inefficient: Two athletes went, then the others. They also didn't meet the standard on one side. Basically, everyone has to be standing on the other side before they go down for the next burpee.

I quickly played with some rep options and then briefed them on the event. I had finalized the rep count just a few minutes before the brief.

#### 3 ROUNDS WITH BODY ARMOR:

#### ONE TRIO RUNS THE COURSE WITH THE LITTER WHILE THE OTHER TRIO DOES 18 BURPEES

#### ROTATE

The timing worked out great. When one group finished the burpees, the other was basically getting in from the litter carry. They repeated this over and over, and the timing continued to play out correctly.

By the third round, I could tell the event was going to be a tad faster than I wanted, so I told them to do a fourth round. *"Really?"* the swimmer snapped at me. I wasn't joking. Julian and Stephane laughed. They know the deal. I guess I forgot to tell her ahead of time how it works. If you are a new tester, hearing that must really suck. They all did the extra round and finished the entire event in 18:39.

They were worked, spent, laid out on the floor. I liked how this one played out, both as a test and as an event. Visually, it's not the best format, but I'll sacrifice that to keep the intensity high and keep people moving. We'll address the visual on site and make sure the correct story is told and that the race is shown in a good way. Working with teams of six is hard. So many bodies moving on the floor. To keep the intensity up, you have to get creative.

After some rest—and some knockout—I briefed them on the new version of the final. The first version we tested had some athletes holding the light Worm while others did rope climbs and handstand push-ups. Then they did a Worm clean complex. Three rounds of that. The new version I'm playing around with has them doing all their gymnastics work and holding in one section. Once finished, they do the Worm complex.

WHILE TEAM HOLDS WORM, PAIRED ATHLETES EACH PERFORM:

I ROPE CLIMB AND IO HSPU

THEN EACH MEMBER OF EACH PAIR PERFORMS:

2 ROPE CLIMBS AND I5 HSPU

THEN EACH MEMBER OF EACH PAIR PERFORMS:

3 ROPE CLIMBS AND 20 HSPU

THEN THE TEAM PERFORMS:

20 WORM COMPLEXES (CLEAN, 2 SQUATS, STEP OVER, REPEAT)

For the rounds of 1 and 10, it took 2 minutes for everyone to cycle through.

For 2 and 15, it took them 3:21.

The round of 3 and 20 took everyone about 6:30, making their total time 11:50 for that portion. The hold in this version is much harder than in the first version. It was a real mental struggle for them. I liked this part of it much better.

On the final part, it took them about a minute to get 5 reps of the complex. That took them to 12:57. The next 5 were finished at 14:28, and they had logged 5 more at 16:22. The final 5 were complete at 18:02. On those last 10 reps, they were really fighting to finish. One male member of the team was breaking down and really struggling, but they fought through. This is a better version. I'm going to think of ways to play with it, and I'll sketch it out on paper and play with the numbers some more before finalizing it.

*Monday, July 24, 10:55 a.m.*

I came into Yarrow this morning. Just working on some last-minute details before I leave on Friday. I feel like it's all coming together now. I took a look at Sunday, and I actually made a huge change to the schedule. I moved the first Individual event before the first Team event. I hadn't planned for that, and I also cut the final Team event to include just the top 10 teams and not 20. That way I can increase the time of that final event to accommodate the version I have now.

Because I'm increasing the time, and after looking at the numbers on paper, I'm making some changes to the event. I'm going to have them do 1 rope climb and 10 handstand push-ups, 2 rope climbs and 20 handstand push-ups, and finally 3 rope climbs and 30 handstand push-ups. For the final section of cleans, I'll have them do 30 instead of 20. All the numbers now play nicely off of each other and make sense in my mind. It will be a great and grueling final test. I'm happy with this version.

This is a huge schedule change late in the game, and major pieces are moving. I don't even know if we can do it because of all the other things already in play, but I'm going to try. I need to check with Justin to see if IT—and the app and everything else—can handle such a big schedule change. We should be fine.

*Tuesday, July 25, 6:42 a.m.*
The schedule change for Sunday wasn't an issue. So I got that cleaned up.

I took a look at the Age Group schedule and saw that they were ending after 7 on Saturday, and I didn't want that to happen. The team pushed back and said that's the best they could do, so last night I spent an hour or so diving into the Age Group schedule and programming for Saturday. I chopped it up so I could get it to end almost an hour earlier. The changes I made involved shortening an event and taking some complexity out of an event. That's necessary to have the day end at a reasonable time while still preserving the needed test of fitness. It's bad enough that our Team and Individual competitions have to go so long, but the Age Group events do not need to go all day, too.

I didn't sleep great last night. I'm starting to feel unsettled, like I should be in Madison already. I don't feel nervous. I just feel ready to be in that environment and in the process of making it all happen. Once I get out there, I'll feel better. But for now I'm itching to be in Madison.

*Wednesday, July 26, 10:08 a.m.*
Today I'm working on lots of last-minute details. I also started my personal packing process. I stopped doing CrossFit.com today. I'm making the transition to lower-intensity workouts so I'm not completely beat up or sore going into the Games. I went for a 3-mile run today, and my mind was all over the map. I was thinking about the week, thinking about announcements I'll have to make, thinking about events in general. My mind will probably be all over the place until I get to Madison.

I really need to be in the chaotic environment that is the Games right now. That's the environment I thrive in. Two more days until I'm there.

In the meantime, I'm going to do a few things here at Yarrow. I'll pack some of the stuff that will go with me and work on the Team Series events. Pat and Stephane wrote them up for me, and now I'm chopping them up. They did a good job, and I'll use 60-75 percent of what they created. But I'm making some changes. I want to see some things done differently for those events. It's annoying to work on them in the middle of the Games, but it needs to be done, so I'm doing it.

Yesterday I posted a pic of the O-course, and people seem very excited about it. Rogue and the team are building the course, and it should be done, or close to being done, by the time I get there on Friday afternoon. I'll probably go straight from the airport to the venue that day.

*Friday, July 28, 8:45 p.m.*

As I was getting ready to board my flight for Madison this morning, I texted Stephane and asked him when the Demo Team shows up. He said they arrive today. "*Perfect,*" I replied. "*I land at 3:45. I am going straight to the venue. Have them there to meet me so we can start testing.*" Time is a precious commodity at this point, and I'm going to maximize what we have. I have no choice. We need to. Once there, front loading becomes very important.

My two flights were easy. I had planned on working on some of the Team Series programming and writing for this book, but I ended up watching the extended director's cut of "*Troy.*" Having recently finished "*The Iliad,*" I was very interested in seeing the movie again. I enjoyed it. It's not exactly like "*The Iliad,*" but it's close enough. I knew a lot of the characters and understood who they were and what they represented because I had just finished the book. The problem is that the director's cut is three hours long, so I didn't finish it on the first leg. By the time I finished watching it on the second leg, I didn't want to dive into CrossFit work. Instead, I picked up the book I'm currently reading, "*Mythology,*" and dove into it for the remainder of the flight. Obviously, "*The Iliad*" influenced this book choice, too.

Upon landing in Madison, I was greeted by the CrossFit Games signage around the airport. It looks good but not great. I think next year we need to step it up a notch or two. Make it over the top.

Once I got my bags and car, I met with Karianne Anthes, my right-hand lady for the week. We went to Starbucks, then to the venue.

Driving into the venue felt great. The signage on the outside of some of the buildings gave it a great feel, like we are here and it is our home. It feels like months and years have built up to this, and it's finally here. The Games are in Madison, and I'm here to make that happen. It feels real now.

We drove straight to where the field and the O-course are set up. The field looks amazing, but I actually laughed: It looks a little small. Don't get me wrong. I'm happy with how it came out, but in terms of scale, I was not overly impressed. That's mostly because the O-course has such a big footprint. The O-course looks like something ripped out of the pages of "*The*

*Iliad*," something Achilles would have had his soldiers run through during the games he put on to celebrate Patroclus' life and death.

As soon as we got out of the car, I said hello to Bill Henniger and some of the crew. Justin and Bill were in good spirits, excited about the course. It felt good to be among them and good to go to work.

The Demo Team was there, and I told them to warm up to run through it with no practice at all. Ben Alderman was the first person to go. He's a big man, and he cruised through it in about 1:43—a good run. On the middle section, he went over the walls and under the logs, which was what we had intended. When I watched him do it, it was underwhelming, so I had the rest of the testers go over the logs instead. In a later section, they crawl under some netting, so having them go under the logs was unnecessary. I liked the speed that small change created.

The Demo Team ladies and some of the other members of the group went through. The ladies did not go sub 2 but were all sub 3.

At first I was kinda flat on the course. I really liked it. I really liked the design. But I guess I was hoping it would be faster. I was hoping they would rip through it, almost like they did at Pendleton, where the times were around 40 seconds. As I was considering all this and looking at ways to speed things up a tad, I noticed everyone else was in love with it. Everyone else was so enthusiastic and felt like it was damn near perfect. I mentally stepped back and reconsidered the course. *"Yeah, it's not Pendleton's course, and that's OK."* It's a little bit slower, and it has different challenges, but that's fine. It has its own unique look, and it definitely does not look like any of the typical OCR shit you see. It has a very hardcore MIL feel to it. That's important to me. Not the hardcore part but the military feel. That keeps it legit and authentic. It's true to my roots and who I am.

We ran a bunch of tests, and then I decided to figure out how the teams would do it. I originally thought of having them do it relay style, but after seeing how long it was taking our guys, I decided to have the whole team go through it as a group. That worked great. Everyone went over the net, across the swing and across the monkey bars, and then team members waited at the wall until everyone else arrived. Then they all finished the rest of the course. It took the team about 4 minutes to do the whole thing that way. I heard Ben say this version was hard, so I liked where it was going.

I had Paul Tremblay do a final run. *"Don't fuck it up—and push it. I want to post this video,"* I told him. He went after it and pushed hard, nailing everything. He ended up finishing in 1:24 or so, the second- or third-fastest time of our testing runs.

I had David Tittle, our camera guy that evening, upload the footage and send it over to me. He's our CrossFit Training media guy, a Level 1 Seminar Staff member and a former CrossFit affiliate owner. While back in my room this evening, I watched it and realized a couple of things. We need to add a section of platform after the rope transfer so that obstacle has natural start and end points. Step on the platform, cross the ropes, step on other platform, come off. Without that last platform, we were having trouble figuring out when an athlete could come off the rope and move to the next obstacle. This addition would solve the problem. I called Bill and asked if that change was possible, and he said no problem.

Another thing I thought about: I wonder if the teams can go down and back. We actually have more time in that window, and I want to use some of it rather than reduce it. I called Justin, and he was still at the venue. I asked him to try running it backward. He did and said it was possible. Tomorrow, I'll have the Demo Team test a down-and-back version.

I took some time to get settled into the hotel. I unpacked all my stuff, had dinner in the room and I started thinking about tomorrow. I can't stop thinking about the O-course and how to have the individuals and teams do it. I actually considered making teams and individuals do it with body armor. I probably won't do that, but I considered it.

Testing in the morning at 9.

*Saturday, July 29, 5:45 a.m.*
I woke up early this morning. I'm going to go the hotel gym, do an easy workout and get some breakfast before heading over to the venue. I haven't made any decisions yet on the running of the O-course. As soon as I show up, I'll have the Demo Team run it twice.

*2:12 p.m.*
We met at the venue at 9 a.m., and I had the team test the O-course down and back. I wanted to see how this version played out relative to others we've tried. It took the team about 3 minutes to get down and then 3 minutes to get back. I had Michael McCoy film it so we can use the video as a teaser, but

it was a very sloppy run. People fell from obstacles and didn't start back at the proper place, and they just generally didn't look so great. But I like the down-and-back plan, and I'm willing to try that out as an option. I discussed it with Justin, Stephane and Todd Widman, and they suggested starting at the end and finishing at what is our beginning—flipping it around. I'm good with that. We'll try that this afternoon with the Demo Team. I'll tell them, *"No falling and do it right."*

After that, we tested the odd-object event. This turned out to be a big moment for me—a moment of disappointment and an opportunity to relearn a good lesson.

I've been planning this event for months: Athletes take the gear halfway across the field, then take it back. In testing at Yarrow, we conducted it like that, and I described it like that in all the briefs to my team. It was set up this way because of logistics: The gear starts where it ends, so there is minimal reset work for our judges and volunteers.

I had Albert-Dominic Larouche do it, and he ended up crushing it. He did it in 6 or 7 minutes, and it was probably the fastest time we've seen in testing. But as I was watching him do it, I realized it was going to be hard to track. It will be confusing and hard to figure out who's winning. I played out multiple scenarios in my mind to see if I could figure out where someone is in the race at any given moment. It was clear there would be a ton of confusion and no clear visual to show who's winning.

I was sitting in the bleachers, and I could see it wasn't working visually. I quickly thought about how we could make it go one length of the field, which would create an entirely better event and race for both the fans and athletes. I called Justin over and said, *"I've made a big mistake, and don't let me do it again."*

*"What's that?"* he asked. I said I should never program Individual events at the Games to cater to logistics or staffing. I should program them to the needs of the competition, to the needs of the athlete, to the needs of the story—then make the logistics work. In this case, that means our staff will have 5 minutes to move one yoke, two farmers-carry handles and a sled across the field—and multiply that by 10 lanes.

We called out J-Mac and spoke to him about it. I told him basically it needs to get done. He said no problem—they will make it happen. That led us to reprogram the event to tell the story better and use the field. After playing around with it, here's what we decided on: Move an object 60 feet north to the middle of the field, handstand-walk 60 feet back to the other objects, move another object 60 feet north to the middle *(leaving it with the other object)*, handstand-walk 60 feet south to the beginning, move the final object 60 feet north to the middle of the field. At this point, all the objects are in the middle of the field. Now we repeat the process, heading north again until all three objects are on the far end of the field. It starts in one end zone and ends in the other.

The big loss here is the reduced amount of handstand walking. We went from 360 total feet of handstand walking to 240. We had a couple of athletes test it this way. The challenge is still there, and the test is still significant. Both Alex Parker and Kelley Jackson did it in around 7 minutes. Alison Scudds struggled with the farmers carries, and we actually stopped her on her last set.

These are big changes, but they're very necessary. All this will make it a much better event. This is another reason why we test events at the CrossFit Games a few days beforehand. We need to understand how they feel, what they look like and where we need to make changes.

After that, we did a bunch of testing with the Big Bob. We had them push, and we had them try something new: pulling it by the handles. The push was fast and the pull was not. Something else we had them do: a little *"suicide course"*—run, push, run, push. It was anticlimactic and didn't really look good. The course is smaller than I had imagined, so it wasn't a good look.

Finally, after some deliberation and rest, we had the team push it the length of the field, turn around and pull it back the length of the field. That took almost 4 minutes, and it looked painful. That might be a good version to do. Justin had suggested having them pull it backward and then push it for the last part, and that's not a bad idea, either. I really want to sign off on it and say it's good right now, but I know the right thing to do is test it a little more. I'm going to go into the schedule and make some changes to the timing for that event.

*9:12 p.m.*
We took a break this afternoon, then had the crew meet up at 3 p.m. for some more testing. We started with the Team O-course, and we had the

athletes start opposite from where the individuals will start. They go down and back. It went well. Alex fell off the bar once, but other than that they had a good, solid run. They finished with a time of about 6:31. This version is good. We'll run with it.

After a short rest we went to the bicycle course. J-Mac briefed them on the bikes and then let them take a little test lap. I hopped on a bike and took a run at the course, too. It's great. It has some good obstacles and sections, and it will be a good test. After 1 lap, my legs were fatigued, and I was feeling the effort.

We then had the Demo Team athletes do a time trial. The fastest of them, Albert, did it in 7:12. The slowest—I think it was Alison—did it in 8:30. Those times are good, and faster than I expected. Before this I was doubting the 3-lap test, but now I think that length will be great. We'll do time trials on Wednesday, followed by the race on Thursday. All this will make for a great expression of this event.

Later that day, we ended up testing the Banger event at its true length.

*Sunday, July 30, 3:34 p.m.*
We got a lot accomplished today. The first thing we did this morning was meet up and have a few of the ladies test the Individual final. The version I've had tested is 3-5-8 reps of handstand push-ups and deadlifts. The men do 5-8-13. Both sexes will perform overhead lunges for 89 feet. I wanted to try having the women do the same reps as the men on the deadlifts. So they would do 5-8-13 deadlifts and 3-5-8 handstand push-ups.

We had Jen Smith test it first. The handstand push-ups challenged her, as we knew they would. If we were to use 5-8-13 reps, it would be really challenging and would slow the event down way too much, affecting our intended stimulus and the time cap. The deadlift section was more challenging than in the original version. The lunges were tough for her. Her total time was 4:40.

Next, we had Kelley do it, and she was able to go a little faster on everything—especially the lunges. She finished right around 4:10.

Albert did it in just under 5 minutes.

All is looking good with this one. I expect 50-65 percent of both the men's and women's fields to finish this test on Sunday.

## AUGUST 2017

*Tuesday, Aug. 1, 8:47 p.m.*

It's been a crazy few days getting around the venue, checking on all aspects of the setup, going over the workouts, meeting with the teams.

I haven't had any time to update this or make entries. Before the Games, I imagined coming back to the computer multiple times throughout the day and at night to update this log. But it's just been too much too fast. I'm moving in too many directions to do that. There are 100 things to do each day. I'll try to make entries when I can, but they won't be a priority. Running the Games is my priority now. There will be a point when I just can't make entries during the event.

First thing yesterday morning, we met a pro cyclist at the cyclocross course and let him take a few runs at it. He did a practice lap, and it was obvious right away that he was a pro. He flew around the course. Then we set him up to do a time trial. He took off flying, and he actually bunny-hopped the logs. When he went over the wood planks, he got off at the last second, ran right over them and then leapt back on the bike. I was blown away by the speed. His total time was 5:30-something. On our Demo Team, our fastest time was 7:20. So the pro was almost 2 minutes faster.

Later in the day, we also tested the Worm/front-squat event—the new version with 40/30 cals and 30 Worm squats. The Demo Team finished it 1:40 over the cap. They were getting worked by the Worm, so we decided to increase the cap by a minute. We're all confident most of the teams can finish it under the cap. Not all, but most. Those changes will be good.

I also checked out the stadium, and it's coming together nicely. The lighting looks amazing, the floor is tight, and the bleachers—the additional ones we added—really make it seem like a gladiatorial arena. The stadium really amps me up for the events it will host.

Last night, I did a little announcement for the Individual athletes. I introduced the clean weights and showed them a video of the cyclocross rider doing the course. I fucked up the weights on the women's side. I tried memorizing them and I was off by 5 lb. for four weights. When I don't have a lot of time to prepare, I have to remember to just use a cheat sheet.

We also had the Individual athletes take a practice run through the O-course. Chelsey Hughes took a big fall on the course. They were flipping over the top of the first obstacle, the cargo net, and she lost her grip and fell almost from the top.

*Wednesday, Aug. 2, 9:20 p.m.*

Today we did the time trials for the bike event—the first event at the 2017 CrossFit Games. It wasn't really the first event because no points were earned, but the trial is important for seeding the races tomorrow.

The course and the event exceeded my expectations. I was really pleased with it and how it played out. I was blown away by some of the times. Ricky Garard cranked out the fastest time at 6:00 flat, and Mat Fraser was a few seconds behind him for the second-fastest time. I didn't see Garard's run, but I saw most of Mat's. Mat was attacking the course the entire time. He had an aggressive posture and was noticeably faster than anyone else in his heat. This raises a question: What can't this guy do?

I saw Josh Bridges struggle on the bike, and his time put him toward the back of the pack. I haven't seen him since then, but he's probably pissed off. Scott Panchik had the slowest time, but he also crashed on the course and his chain came off, so he had to deal with those delays.

On the women's side, Kristin Holte had the fastest time. Her 6:45 was faster than 15 of the men. Sam Briggs was second. I was very impressed by how she attacked the course, too. Some of the athletes looked hungry and aggressive, and others looked passive and confused. Brooke Wells really struggled, as did Camille Leblanc-Bazinet. I saw Brooke on the course, and she looked very uncomfortable. I heard she fell four times, but I didn't see any of that.

What's interesting is that the athletes have experienced versions of a couple of the events and have time to think about them before we start scoring. Yesterday, they did the O-course, and if they struggled, they now have time to think about that and worry about it.

*Monday, Aug. 14, 4:59 p.m.*
It's been about a week since the Games ended. Eight days exactly.

I've avoided this project for a few reasons: exhaustion from the event and disinterest.

In the days immediately following the event, I wasn't really interested in talking about it or writing down my thoughts. Even as I write now, I don't know if I'm really into it. I feel like putting it off. But this task is also haunting me right now.

I spent months preparing for the Games. Then they came and went in four days, and this project feels like the last unfinished part of the Games.

This final section starts with disappointment.

At the end of the event, I was happy it was over, but I was also disappointed—in myself, primarily. Some things we did, things I oversaw, did not go as planned. There were a number of contributing factors. No single thing specifically disappointed me, but a number of small things left me feeling unhappy. I'm very critical of what we do, what I do, and what the team does. When things aren't almost perfect, it's easy for me to be disappointed.

I've painted a picture of disappointment, but let me be clear: The Games were a huge success. The staff, the volunteers, Rogue, Reebok—we all came together. We put on a great event, and we used a great test that truly determined the Fittest on Earth: Mat Fraser and Tia-Clair Toomey.

For the most part, the things that upset me didn't affect that test or the spectacle. The best way for me to close this off is to dive into each event and review what happened each day. That's how I'll handle this book from here. The following sections were written from mid-August to early September as I reflected on what happened during the Finals.

*Day 1 of the Games—Thursday, Aug. 3*
Thursday was the first of four days of competition. It was the first time we had a four-day competition like this. In the early years, it was usually two or three days. When we went to four days of competition in 2012, it was one day on, one day off and three days on. Last year, the individuals actually competed for five days straight, but Thursday, Day 2, had a swim event and nothing else, so it was very low impact and not demanding at all. I obviously

programmed it that way so it was like a rest day for them because of the demands of the trip to Aromas the day before.

Having done this four-day event this way, I think I want to go back to Wednesday on, Thursday off and then Friday to Sunday on. From the standpoint of the organizer and the event team, this schedule gives everyone a day to work hard, a day to reset and prep, and then a three-day push instead of a four-day push. This plan will also keep the fans fresh and excited, and it will give the athletes a day of recovery that will allow them to attack the final three days of competition hard.

I'm not unhappy with how the four-day competition went. I think it was good. It was necessary to try it out in our development of this grand sport. The athletes could handle it, but I feel like the one-on, one-off, three-on schedule will be something we do next year.

I showed up very early on Thursday morning before Run Swim Run. I went to the start and checked everything out. It all looked good. Then I talked to Justin, and we decided to check out the water and the turnaround. We got out there about 45 minutes before the event started, and it was a complete shit show. Things were just getting set up, and most of the infrastructure we needed wasn't in place.

I was baffled. Here we are on Day 1 of the CrossFit Games, and the course for our first event isn't set up 30 minutes before it starts. Barricades were being set, signage was being put out, placards were being laid out, and I was standing there perplexed.

Given the demands of my role as Director of the Games, other people run certain special projects and events. This is due to the scale of the CrossFit Games. I can't run every little thing—nor should I. In this case, our lead basically decided to set up the course at the last minute, and the team was rushing to make it happen.

I was furious. I barked a few commands and yelled at a few people on my team. I was just blown away that this was happening. It was poor planning, and it looked horrible. We were about 15 minutes from the start, and I needed to get back to the main campus for that. Justin said he would stay and oversee the work at the turnaround, and I zipped back to the start.

A few minutes before the event kicked off, Justin called and told me it was all set. I was slightly relieved, but not much.

As is customary, I counted down and kicked off the first event. It was pouring rain by the time they took off. I loved the rain, and I loved the dreariness. I love having the athletes do these tests in less-than-ideal situations. This type of weather really showcases character and grit and separates those who will fight from those who won't.

### CROSSFIT GAMES INDIVIDUAL EVENT I: RUN SWIM RUN

### RUN I.5 MILES

### SWIM 500 M

### RUN I.5 MILES

The athletes took off at a blistering pace. I followed closely on my bicycle for the first half-mile or so, then took a shortcut across the field to get in front of the pack. I rode in front of the group by a few hundred yards for a few reasons: to make sure the course was clear and marked and to keep track of what was going on in the front.

I got to the water, and I think Mat Fraser was the first there, followed closely by Brent Fikowski. They both entered the water, and then everyone else showed up and started getting in the water, too. I watched the water portion until the first athlete—Fikowski—got out. Then I got on my bike and headed back to the start.

Everything was set for them to run across the finish line. It was still pouring rain, and a ton of fans were there. Fikowski came around the corner, and on the last stretch Tia-Clair Toomey and Kristi Eramo were running right behind him. They almost passed him to take the overall win, and I was very impressed by that. Tia-Clair and Kristi were only beaten by Fikowski. They beat every other male athlete in the field in an event that was exactly the same for everyone. They all came in around 28:45.

When we had Chase Ingraham test it, he was in the low 30s. When we talked about the test afterward, we agreed some people would be just under 30 and most would be around the low 30s. As it played out, three women were under 30 minutes, five were in the 30-31 range, and the rest were over 31. Alethea Boon was slowest, at more than 41 minutes.

I noted how Katrin Davidsdottir did. She was 14th, and I thought she would have done much better given how much she trains with endurance coach Chris Hinshaw and how much she runs. Brooke Wells finished 16th. That's a huge improvement from a year ago when she almost finished last on the run event in Aromas. I think her Run Swim Run placing came at a cost, though.

On the men's side, Brent was in at 28:45, and about 30 seconds later Jonne Koski came in. Koski was a national-champion swimmer, and he's always done well in the swim events at the Games, so that made sense. I was pleased to see Ben Smith come in third. It was a nice way for him to start the Games. Mat came in seventh.

Eight men were under the 30-minute mark, and 10 were between 30 and 31 minutes. The slowest male, Michael Palomba, finished at 44:30, more than 3 minutes slower than the slowest female. I don't know if Palomba had some issues or what. I never followed up.

I think the biggest surprise for me was Josh Bridges coming in 32nd, at 33:43. Josh has traditionally been great at the swim and run events at the Games. His background as a SEAL and his ability to run fast give him a great advantage in those events. But here he ends up finishing 32nd on Run Swim Run with a time that also put him behind 25 females.

I had this event start at 8 a.m. sharp, and the Team event was to start at 9 a.m. sharp. That's how the schedule had it. That's how I planned it. That was the plan from the beginning. At about 8:55, Chuck, my lead judge for the teams, comes up and says he's being told by the broadcast truck that the start is going to be a few minutes after 9.

The days leading up to the competition had been full of frustrating scheduling issues. On Tuesday and Wednesday, we had big meetings in which I learned pieces of the schedule were wrong. Wrong based on what? Wrong based on what I created. As you know from this book, I put a lot of time and effort into the schedule, and I consider every single minute and detail of each event. The schedule, to me, is part of the art that is this event.

What happened was a few people on the team thought it would be harmless to add a few minutes here and there. The problem is I have the master schedule, and I know where and when everything is. Everything falls out of place when minutes are added in different places. We spent way too much time fixing the schedule in the days leading up to the event. That time should not have been spent there, but we had to do it because of the errors that were created.

Come Thursday morning, I expected everything to be straight on the schedule. Yet before the second event of the morning, I hear we need to start at a time that's different from what I had on the schedule. I was pissed, as you can imagine. I told Chuck to tell them no: *"We are starting the event at 9 a.m. exactly."*

The last individual came in at 8:44, so the teams had 16 minutes before 9—plenty of time. We got them set, and it was still raining. At 9 a.m. exactly, they took off.

The day before the event, I made a change to fix the order. Originally, I had it so they could choose any order they wanted, but then I decided a change would make it easier to control and easier to follow. We had them use a male pair first, a female pair second and then a mixed pair for the third and final leg.

### 2017 CROSSFIT GAMES TEAM EVENT I: RUN SWIM RUN

RELAY AS PAIRS (MM, FF, MF):

RUN 1.5 MILES

SWIM 500 M

RUN 1.5 MILES

As the teams took off, I followed closely behind on my bike. I rode out with the first group, and then I rode ahead of them to make it to the water first. Once I got to the staging area, I looked around and noticed signage was missing and things were not in place. The signage was fucked up again, and the event was already underway. Some teams had name placards and others didn't. To be fair, most had name placards, but a few didn't. Placards were critical because team members were briefed to place their gear on their name placards.

The first day of the CrossFit Games in a new location was not going well.

Our team and the other teams handled the issue well, and it didn't affect the competition.

I rode back with the lead group to the start, and when I got there every single remaining team member was on the course in the transition zones. Another frustration. I pulled Chuck aside and asked him why it was that way. It wasn't what we had talked about or what I had briefed. He had a reason, but it wasn't strong enough and I didn't like it. So before the first pairs showed up to transition, I sent all the final pairs back into the beer garden to stage. The beer garden is where we had the teams set up for the event.

All this led to more frustration on my part. I felt like I was losing control. I wasn't, but I had to take a few deep breaths to calm myself down. After watching the transition go down a few times for the teams, I told Chuck he had the event. I needed to leave for the cyclocross event that was going to start in less than an hour.

Overall, I was happy with how Run Swim Run went. It was a good course, and it had the desired effect on everyone.

Later in the day, during the Age Group competition, apparently a masters athlete who was on the verge of drowning was saved by another athlete. We published a story on the event, but later on the athlete who was saved said it didn't really happen that way and wanted us to pull the story. I still don't know what the truth is or what really happened, but I'm glad nobody died on the swim.

The turnaround time for the Individual athletes after Run Swim Run was minimal. We had the first Cyclocross heats starting at 10 a.m. The course was all set, and I showed up ready to tackle something that was going to go down flawlessly. And in terms of behind-the-scenes issues and logistics, it basically was flawless.

We brought the first heat out and started the race on time. A ton of fans were there. I don't know how many, but I was really surprised at how many showed up. More and more spectators showed up as the heats proceeded.

### 2017 CROSSFIT GAMES INDIVIDUAL EVENT 2: CYCLOCROSS

### 3 LAPS OF CYCLOCROSS COURSE

I thought the races were really good and the event was running smoothly. We actually bumped up the heats and finished some of them ahead of schedule because we had the flexibility to do that. In an event like this, I like to think of the schedule as dynamic. If we have room to compress, we compress. If not, we stay on schedule. Here, we had a lot of room to compress, so we did.

There were some accidents and some passes in great races. Mat Fraser impressed me again, but the real star on the male side was Ricky Garard. He finished first in 19:26, and Mat was second with a time of 19:52.

Ricky, I would later learn, grew up riding motorcycles and bikes, and he told me he actually raced flat track at one point, so he obviously understood corners and turns. On the day we did time trials, Ricky had the fastest lap: 6 flat. The day before, we had the pro Trek rider do the course, and his time on one lap was just under 5:40—only 20 seconds faster than Ricky's 6:00. The pro had clip-in pedals, while Ricky did not. GPP at the highest levels translates to some impressive feats. Ricky impressed me on this event, and he would go on to impress me repeatedly.

On the female side, Kristin Holte barely beat Sam Briggs. Holte's 21:43 would have ranked her 20th on the male side.

I liked that event, and I liked the three-lap version of it. Johnny Mac had set up the course and created it from top to bottom. I tasked him with that project months ago, and he ran with it and crushed it. I really liked the course he created: It was great for our athletes. We actually created quite the buzz in the cyclocross world. Fans and athletes of the sport were excited that we included this test.

I was unhappy with some decisions we made and some decisions I made. We had time trials to place athletes in the heats by ability. In the original version, we had 1-20 in one heat and 21-40 in another. Someone on the team suggested a change, and we ended up doing this: Athletes 1-5 from the time trials were in the front row of Heat 1 on race day, and 6-10 were in the first row of the second heat. So basically the top 10 athletes from the time trials were in the first rows of two different race-day heats. I think we would have had better races if we had stuck to the original plan to have 1-20 in one heat and 21-40 in the other. That was a mistake, and I could see it during the heats. In the same heats, some groups of riders were fast and others were slow. I would rather have seen all the fast riders together. Really, though, this is a good learning point for future years.

The other thing we did wrong with this event was the stagger. Before we did the time trial on Wednesday, we heard murmurings from athletes who were planning on sandbagging the time trial because it didn't really matter, so we decided to create a 10-yard stagger between the lines of athletes on race day. The first five athletes were set in a line, and then 10 yards behind them we set the next five. Another 10 yards behind them, we set the next five, followed by the final five another 10 yards back. So the last group was 30 yards from the first, which seemed to be too great a distance for people to make up. As I watched a lot of the races, it seemed like the top five were racing each other most of the time, and those in the next groups were fighting a hard battle to get to them. This procedure did make the time trials really important, but it didn't create as much mass chaos and racing in the front as I was hoping for on race day. I don't know if it's true that those in the second or third rows never made it into the top five. That's something I'll have someone on our team research. It would be interesting to know.

Other than those two things, I wouldn't have changed much. Actually, I might have added a few more obstacles at various points. I think there could have been an additional section of walls to hop over and one or two additional sections of logs to navigate. I was happy with the sand section.

One note: Camille Leblanc-Bazinet came across the finish line in complete tears. I knew she had come into the competition with some shoulder injury. I asked her what was going on, and she said she dislocated her shoulder in a crash on the course but put it back in position during the event. After I briefed the next test, the injury took her out of the Games.

After the event was done, and once the teams were done with Run Swim Run, we gathered all the athletes in the briefing room at the convention center. There, I briefed them on the final Individual and Team events for that evening. It was Amanda .45 for the individuals and Muscle-Up Snatch for the teams. The individuals seemed very excited about it, as did the teams. I don't think they were expecting the increase in reps. They might have been expecting increased weight—that's typically what people do these days with that event—but not increased reps.

### 2017 CROSSFIT GAMES TEAM EVENT 2: MUSCLE-UP SNATCH

MEN COMPLETE 30-24-18-12-6 REPS OF:

MUSCLE-UPS

SQUAT SNATCHES (135 LB.)

THEN WOMEN COMPLETE 27-21-15-9-3 REPS OF:

MUSCLE-UPS

SQUAT SNATCHES (95 LB.)

The Team event was up first in the evening, and it was pretty straight-forward. I actually don't watch much of the actual competition during Team events. I'm watching to make sure the flow is working and the movement is all playing out correctly. I was mostly very happy with how this one went down. At one point, I saw a judge make a mistake on the number of reps a team had to do at a station and call them back incorrectly. I got into Chuck's ear on that one.

The five-station rig I had Rogue build for this event was incredible. It looked amazing, and it was built so all the steel didn't obstruct the sight lines. Justin had actually pushed back on the five-station rig and didn't want to do it, but it was something I said I would not waver on, and I told him to trust me. After the event, he admitted I was right and said it looked great.

I was surprised that Mayhem's men didn't win their section. They took fifth. The Invictus men actually won this event with a time of 10:17. Interestingly, the Wasatch men took 26th, but their women took first with a time of 9:10.

The reps were different for each gender, and, in hindsight, I think this was the right call. Even with that time disparity between the top men and women, the times look a little more similar once you start going down the leaderboard. At 10th, the men's team was at 10:56, while the females were at 10:20. At 20th, the men logged 11:14, and the women finished in 10:56. At 30th, the men completed it in 11:55, and the females took 11:38.

It's always interesting going from the teams to individuals on similar events. We went from having 60 athletes with multiple judges to just 10 total athletes on the floor. It feels like a huge weight is lifted and the event will be easy to conduct because of the reduced numbers.

2017 CROSSFIT GAMES INDIVIDUAL EVENT 3: AMANDA .45

13-11-9-7-5 REPS OF:

MUSCLE-UPS

SQUAT SNATCHES (135/95 LB.)

I thought this event played out great. The races were very obvious, and the finishes were good. The five different rigs and five sets of barbells per athlete helped create clear races and clear visuals of who was winning.

Dakota Rager, a rookie, posted the fastest men's time: 8:01. Had Mat been in his heat, I imagine Mat would have won. Mat was in the final heat, which he won with a time of 8:17. Had Mat been behind someone in his heat, I think he could have pulled off the overall win. Light guys Logan Collins and Cody Anderson were both in the top five, as was Ricky Garard.

Another early big surprise: Josh Bridges finished 18th. I thought for sure this was something he would manhandle, but he appeared to struggle early on.

On the female side, rookie Jamie Greene posted an impressive time of 8:51. Tia-Clair Toomey was second at 8:58, and Emily Bridgers had the third-fastest time: 9:08. Once again, I was surprised at how Katrin did. She finished 24th with 11:50. Brooke Wells finished 33rd. She was 35th in Cyclocross, and her first day was not ending on a positive note.

After seeing all the heats, I realized my time cap was too generous. I had a 17-minute cap for the women and a 15-minute cap for the men. I could have used a 12-minute cap for everyone. If we had done 12 minutes, one male would have been capped and 13 females would have been capped. Maybe a 13-minute cap would have been better for the females. Regardless, a tighter cap would have been OK—actually preferable.

While we were inside, a huge storm was battering our campus outside. At one point, we actually had to clear everyone out of the tents and structures and tell them to take cover in the hard structures. I didn't know this was going on until Justin came up to me and said he needed to go outside and check on the Compex booth, which had collapsed.

I stayed in the Coliseum watching over the competition for about five minutes, and then I left to go check on it myself. As reported, it had collapsed. There it lay between the Rogue tent and the FitAID booth. The Compex booth had come down and was completely destroyed. This year, these were really big structures with trusses—large build-outs, not small 10-by-10 or 20-by-20 tents. Luckily, our team had a good plan in place to get people to safe areas when the weather became too severe, and that literally saved lives here.

Impressively, they had another building company come in, take the downed booth away and put up a new one overnight. The next day, they were operating in the booth as if nothing had happened.

That night, I got the team together, and we had a brief talk about the day and some of the mistakes. Then we had a long meeting to go over the plan one more time to make sure everything would be correct the next day.

One day down, three more to go.

*Day 2 of the Games—Friday, Aug. 4*
I woke up around 5 a.m. to the thought of athletes falling from the top of the cargo net as they raced over it, as a few had done in the practice runs.

This morning, we would do the obstacle course. In practice a few days earlier, we had allowed them to do a flip over the top. The flip was very athletic and very fast. It also had severe consequences: falls from a significant height. A few athletes fell from the top, and I even posted one on my Instagram account. Luckily, nobody was injured.

Athletes climbed to the top of the net, then folded at the waist over the log that sits on the top. They reached down as far they could and grabbed the cargo net, then pulled their bodies over the log and flipped their bodies around their hands to a position where their backs were against the cargo net. From there, most just bounced off the net and landed on their feet. Some fucked this part up and caught their feet, which led them to go headfirst into the ground. Others fucked up the flip part and lost their grip. Either way, I realized a few things on that practice day: The flip was going to be the fastest technique by far, and if an athlete didn't use the technique, he or she was not going to advance or be competitive.

It had been raining the day before, and it was dreary and wet on Friday morning. I had these horrible visions of the athletes using that technique because they essentially had to, with some falling to horrible results. I called Boz and Justin to my room at the hotel, and I told them I was going to change it. I was going to require them to throw one leg over the top log and then the other, so they have to crawl over the top in a controlled manner. We already were going to implement this rule for the Team and Age Group athletes, and we decided to apply it to the individuals, too.

Justin and Boz pushed back a little. They thought it was fine to let the individuals flip, but because of the wet conditions and the fact that the weather wasn't supposed to improve, I stayed with the decision. (*Sitting here a few weeks later, I firmly believe that was the right call.*)

Nobody got hurt falling from the cargo net. If we had let them flip, it's possible no one would have fallen and been hurt, but it wasn't worth the risk.

### 2017 CROSSFIT GAMES INDIVIDUAL EVENT 4: SPRINT O-COURSE

#### OBSTACLE-COURSE RACE

I was very happy with how the event played out. It was great. It was very different from the one we did in Pendleton. At first, I struggled with that, but then after having athletes test it and understanding what we had, I was pleased with it. I even came to really like how different it was from the Pendleton obstacle course we used in 2012.

The first heats took what felt like a long time to get through, but it really wasn't. We had to run heats of five, so it took eight heats to get everyone through so we could determine the advancing athletes. We had one athlete—I think it was Tommy Vinas—do a borderline flip over the top of the cargo net, and we gave him a stiff warning not to do it again or he would be disqualified. Alec Smith got no repped coming over the net for touching the black line that was out of bounds. That took him out of contention. He was thought to be a favorite going in because of his gymnastics ability and athleticism.

At the end of all the preliminary male heats, we had five athletes for the final: Patrick Vellner, Streat Hoerner, Cody Anderson, Noah Ohlsen and Jonne Koski. Cody and Noah had both impressed me in earlier heats, and I thought they might win. Patrick had struggled in one of his preliminary heats, but he came through strong and took the win to get 100 points. Mat Fraser ended up sixth. Yet more surprises: Josh Bridges was 19th, and Brent Fikowski, a big favorite, finished eighth.

The weather was still cold, wet and gloomy for the women. It was, in my eyes, perfect. I loved that weather and I loved that it rolled in on us for the o-course.

The women were slightly slower than the men. The course was identical for them, but they are, generally speaking, a bit smaller than the men. But the women's side of the event was no less exciting. We saw some great races, some near misses and some close finishes.

For the final heat, Tennil Reed-Beuerlein, Anna Tobias, Annie Thoris-dottir, Bethany Branham and Katrin Davidsdottir raced against each other. Tennil took the win and 100 points for this event. She was on her way to a great Games performance. Brooke Wells finished 37th, which was dead last with three athletes out of the competition. She really struggled on this event. Tia-Clair took 12th.

## 2017 CROSSFIT GAMES TEAM EVENT 3: TEAM O-COURSE

### OBSTACLE-COURSE RACE

We cleared the individuals and switched gears for the team competition. We had Team athletes go down and back, and at certain points they had to stop and wait for their teammates before proceeding. They had 8 minutes to do it. The Demo Team had done this exact test in 6 minutes, so I figured 8 was plenty. I was wrong.

After a few heats, no teams had finished it, and I was becoming worried that not a single team would finish. Eventually one team finished it, and by the end a total of eight teams had finished. I'm really happy some teams finished, and I would have been disappointed if they had all hit the time cap. (*That disappointment would come later.*)

12 Labours CrossFit had the fastest time: 6:37. Wasatch was fourth in 6:47. Mayhem tied for ninth but didn't finish the course.

My intent in programming this one was to have more teams finish. I would have liked at least half the field or more to finish. That didn't happen, and it's a good learning point. Sometimes the Demo Team will be much better than other teams, so I need to buffer testing times, especially on something as odd and unique as an O-course.

At 12:30 p.m., we had 30 minutes before the Team Clean and Jerk started. We moved into the stadium and saw the floor laid out with the weights and platforms. It looked great wide open. The day before, we had the five gigantic rigs on the floor, and today the floor was 90 percent open. In programming the Games, I take the appearance into consideration, too. Some days the floor is cluttered with rigs, and other days it's wide open.

Generally speaking, I like to end on Sunday with a wide-open floor. Of late, we haven't always done that.

## 2017 CROSSFIT GAMES TEAM EVENT 4/5: CLEAN AND JERK (F AND M)

### 1-REP-MAX CLEAN AND JERK

The Team clean and jerk was pretty straightforward in terms of execution. Not a lot to go wrong. The one thing that's not ideal is that it's not super easy to tell who's winning or who's lifting big. We do have signage to show what people will lift, so that helps. And our announcers for the teams, Larry Moss and Josh Gallegos, did a great job of focusing the crowd on the big lifts—and we had some of those. Some Team athletes were gigantic, and it actually looked as if some of them grew in stature for this event.

I remember seeing a few people go for 400 lb. I think one got it, but I'm not sure. I also remember seeing one of the strongest team members using a power clean and push jerk! CrossFit 417 ended up winning the male portion. The team total was 1,054 lb., meaning their average lift per male athlete was 351 lb.

Austin Malleolo, Spencer Hendel and Conor Murphy of Reebok CrossFit One took fourth with 1,001 lb. CrossFit Mayhem took 10th with a total of 978 lb. I knew going in Rich had some knee issues. (*At the time of writing after the Games on Aug. 16, I texted back and forth with him, and yesterday he had knee surgery to fix both knees. Hopefully he makes a quick recovery from that.*)

On the female side of the house, Salt Lake City CrossFit had the biggest total: 698 lb., for an average of 232 per athlete. That's really impressive. NorCal CrossFit Redwood City lifted 684 lb. to finish third, and Wasatch CrossFit tied for ninth overall. Mayhem's women finished 21st. Up until that point, the team's lowest finish in five events was 10th, so 21st really hurt.

I was happy once the Team portion of this event was over. Again, this event is not hard to run, but there are so many bodies on the floor and so many moving parts that it's loud and something could go wrong.

The format we used for the Individual athletes was going to make their lifting—snatching—exciting.

## 2017 CROSSFIT GAMES INDIVIDUAL EVENT 5: 1RM SNATCH

### 1-REP-MAX SNATCH

We used a format in which a different athlete lifted every 20 seconds, and we rotated through everyone twice. The huge benefit of this format is that everybody is drawn to one lifter. The fans and the broadcast team do not miss a single moment of action. We had three heats, and the top 10 got two additional lifts in a final heat.

The first round was very exciting. All the athletes were looking around to see what the big lifts would be. If you were strong, you had to see what the other strong guys were doing so you could plan and try to advance. If you were not in that category, well, then you had to just lift as much as you could to try and keep your rank high relative to the others who would not advance.

Jeff Patzer had the lowest lift: 225 lb. That seems really low. I'm not sure if he just struggled during the event, but I imagine his 1RM is higher than that. Josh Bridges hit 242 lb., which I know is a lot for him. But that score only placed him 36th.

Higher up, you had athletes such as Alec Smith, Scott Panchik and Alex Anderson all miss the cut to advance, which is surprising because they are all traditionally strong on the Olympic lifts.

After his first round, Tommy Vinas had lifted close to 300, and the announcer asked him about his intent for the second round. *"To lift three blues,"* Vinas replied with the utmost confidence. I loved it, and I was hoping he would lift 315 lb., but he ended up hitting 302 lb. and taking second. To my surprise, Garret Fisher won the event with a 305-lb. lift. I knew Garret was strong, and he's one of the larger athletes in the field, but I just didn't see him winning this event. Mat was fifth with a solid 291, and Ben Smith was right behind him with 290 lb.

On the female side, there was a little more drama in the final heat. I was really surprised to see Brooke Wells not advance to the final. She actually finished tied for 11th with a 187-lb. lift. I view her as one of the stronger athletes in the field, but she didn't crack the top 10. In the final heat you had some other strong females, such as Kara Webb, Alessandra Pichelli, Sara Sigmundsdottir, Annie Thorisdottir, Katrin Davidsdottir and Tia-Clair Toomey.

On the first of two rounds in the final heat, Katrin made an attempt and totally bailed out. She pulled the bar and shrugged but didn't even attempt to drop under or do anything else. I actually thought for a minute that maybe this was her strategy. She's been known to strategize events and sandbag things with an eye on the bigger picture. A few years ago when she won, she took it easy on the pegboard so she could blast the handstand event that came right after. Her decision to do that was very controversial.

Five women ended up lifting 200 lb. or more: Cassidy Lance-McWherter, Sara, Alessandra, Tia and Kara.

Alessandra hit 207 lb. and won the event in dramatic fashion. Katrin missed both her lifts in the final, and I think I saw her leaving the floor in tears, so that made me rethink my theory that she was sandbagging the first lift.

A few minutes after the event was over, Boz came over and said he thought Alessandra's weights were wrong. Someone had a picture of her bar, and it was loaded unequally. She actually only had 202 on it, and it was uneven. But she still hit that lift. We had to adjust the scores, and this gave Kara Webb the event win at 203 lb. Tia tied for second with Pichelli at 202.

Alessandra's loading mistake is hers and her judge's. The athlete is responsible for loading the weight and declaring the load, but I wish the judge would have caught the error and told her the weight was off. We fixed it fast and moved on. No need to dwell on a mistake like that.

I was very happy with how the snatch played out. Max-out events are always a favorite, so this one was hard to mess up. The format in which they lift one at a time was not new, but giving the top 10 lifters an additional 2 lifts was new, and I think it worked out great. We were able to do all the men's heats in one hour, with another hour for the women. The format is a keeper. Maybe it will return next year to the Games or even to Regionals. Actually, not Regionals. It's a Games-only format.

## 2017 CROSSFIT GAMES TEAM EVENT 6: ROWING WORM

### 3 ROUNDS OF:

### 40/30-CAL. ROW (EACH)

### 30 WORM SQUATS

We tested a version of this at Yarrow with fewer reps. From that test, I decided we needed to do a beefed-up version with more reps. Once we got to Madison, we had the Demo Team test it with the new rep scheme. They did not finish: They were actually about a minute over the cap of 12 minutes. But we decided not to change it. With that in mind, I was OK with this event being hard for teams to finish. I was expecting only the best to finish, and that was the case. Only 13 of 40 teams beat the time cap. I was pleased: That was the intent. I think the work was very hard, and people looked blasted afterward.

This was probably the most rowers we've ever had on the floor: 60. Actually, that's not true. We had 80 rowers on the floor in 2013, when we did the half-marathon for the individuals.

Wasatch CrossFit won this one with a time of 10:23. Timberwolf CrossFit was second in 10:30, and Mayhem was third with a time of 10:31. For a Team event, it was pretty straightforward and clean in terms of presentation and how they moved the Worm. I was happy with how it played out.

### 2017 CROSSFIT GAMES INDIVIDUAL EVENT 6: TRIPLE-G CHIPPER

100 PULL-UPS

80 GHD SIT-UPS

60 ONE-LEGGED SQUATS, ALTERNATING

40-CAL. ROW

20 DUMBBELL PUSH PRESSES (100/70 LB.)

I had tested this event numerous times and changed it often. Toward the end of the chipper's creation, a few days before leaving for the Games, I had decided to up the reps to the numbers we used at the Games: 100 pull-ups, 80 GHDs, 60 pistols, 40 calories on the Concept2 rower and 20 push presses. I did that to stretch the time out to the range of 12-14 minutes. The changes ended up stretching it out a little, but not for the top guys and gals. They crushed it.

The top male and top female times make for an interesting comparison. Mat had the top male time: 10:46, about 1:15 faster than what I was expecting the top time to be. Kara Webb had the top female time: 10:45, within a second of Mat's time. The winners were the only athletes to go under 11:00. Second fell to Jamie Greene with 11:04, and to Jonne Koski for the men in 11:05. After that, the comparisons stop. Eight men did it under 12 minutes, and four women were under 12:00. Seventeen men were in the 12-minute range, and eight women were in the 12 range. A total of 25 women took more than 13 minutes, and three of them were capped, including Emily Abbott and Lauren Fisher. I would not have expected that from either one. On the men's side, the athletes from 26th to 39th were over 13 minutes, and only Garret Fisher hit the cap. So he went from winning the snatch event to finishing dead last in the event immediately following.

Those times make me think I accomplished what I wanted: something in the range of 12-14 minutes for most athletes. The best excelled and set very fast times. That's the nature of the sport.

In this event, I carried over something from Regionals: heats of 20, two heats of each gender. We were able to do that because no barbells were in play and each piece of equipment fit within the confines of what is essentially a 5-foot-wide lane. We had Bill create a rig that would accommodate heats of 20.

I'm really glad we did it this way, and I'll try to create more events in which we have heats of 20 at Regionals and the Games. Doing so will speed up the event and the competition overall, and it will tell the story faster, making it easier to follow and more exciting for the fans. This will help us avoid spectator fatigue. Watching the same heats over and over—especially in the really long events—is a drag on spectators.

Overall, I'm happy with how this one came out, especially with all the revisions it went through.

We had a quick 34-minute break, during which I introduced the final Individual event for the night. I had the Rogue team wheel out a banger, which was covered up. I unveiled it, and everyone was excited. I was excited. The announcement was good. I was happy with it, and we had a lot of momentum going into the event. We'd had a good day of competition, and we had a good final test to end the day.

### 2017 CROSSFIT GAMES INDIVIDUAL EVENT 7: ASSAULT BANGER

#### 40/30-CAL. ASSAULT BIKE

#### 20-FT. BANGER

Then it went south.

When the first heat of athletes came out, I immediately noticed that not one was wearing gloves. At that moment I realized we had forgotten to pass out gloves. Our plan was to provide the athletes with gloves they could use if they wanted to. 5.11 Tactical had supplied gloves, but we forgot to get them to the athletes.

The breakdown happened at a few levels, but ultimately I blame myself for the mistake. Months ago, I had requested gloves from 5.11. Multiple people on the team were brought into the loop. In the week leading up to the Games, I asked for the gloves, but they were not there yet. Finally, I got a text from Mason Snyder, our CrossFit POC with 5.11, who said he had the gloves. This was midweek. I forgot to follow up to make sure we had the gloves. A few other people on the team also forgot to check where the gloves were and why we didn't have them. But in the end, I blame myself.

Once the first heat was going, I knew there was nothing we could do. I went to the back during the first heat, and I saw Kurtis Bowler and the Athlete Control team scrambling and asking the Rogue crew to get some gloves. But at that point, it was already too late. We couldn't outfit only some heats with gloves. I was very, very worried hands were going to get torn up and ripped. As the athletes in the first heat were coming off, I checked their hands. Their grip was shot, as expected, but for the most part their hands were OK. A few had small tears, but I was happy to see very little hand damage. After every heat, I watched closely to see how bad their hands were.

Some athletes, such as Mat Fraser, had gloves with them, so they used them. I actually wonder if Mat sent someone to get gloves for him. I only say that because we briefed that event and didn't let them go back to their warm-up area in the convention center. They had to stay underneath the stadium and wait.

That was my first disappointment with this event. The second disappointment was the actual event. In our testing sessions, we had figured out you need to stand even with the front edge of the Banger or slightly in front of it for best contact. We saw something different from almost all the male athletes in the first few heats. The fastest times were coming from those who were standing well behind the front of the block, near the middle of the object. Instead of using a clean strike to drive the block, they were essentially pulling it back with the hammer. There wasn't much we could do, and the fastest time was posted by someone who did this.

Mat Fraser struck cleanly and put all his effort into doing it right, and he was 20th—his lowest placing in the Games. George Sanchez put up the fastest male time: 1:48. Apparently he's a beast on the Assault bike. He cranked his 40 calories out in around 40 seconds, then came off and used the drag technique. I actually didn't see him do it, but multiple people told me he did. George went on to finish the Games 22nd overall.

On the female side, Sam Briggs won in 2:33. Sam is a former firefighter, so her success made sense. She also used the suspect technique, not as blatantly as some people, but subtly—even though I had briefed all the women on where to stand and how to strike prior to their heats. The women's heats looked much better, but some athletes were still using that cheating technique, and our judges were on them more aggressively than they were on the men. Brooke Wells finished that event in 4:28 to take 28th. She came off the floor saying she hit her finger, and a few days after the competition, she posted on Instagram that she had broken her finger during the Games.

That was not the ending I was hoping for on Friday. Essentially, I alone take the blame for the problems. I should have done more testing on that odd object and figured out that you could game and cheat it. But in all the tests we did do, we never came across that technique as an option. When we last used the Banger—in 2012—we had one section of track set at waist height, and some athletes used the push technique there. But on this version with the athletes standing overtop, I didn't think it was going to be an issue at all.

We went into our final meeting on Friday night, and I was discouraged by what had happened with the Banger. Some of Thursday's mishaps were still lingering, too. Not a great start to the Games. It was also not a great start for me, and I was not meeting my own expectations. For the fans and the athletes, the competition was running great. But I hold myself and my team to high standards, and we shouldn't have messed up like this.

As we were going over the Saturday plan, Justin approached me and said, "*We need to make a big change to the schedule.*" Basically, we needed to move the Yelawolf concert to after the competition. We had originally planned to have it during one of our large breaks. This was a huge schedule change, and it baffled me. We were essentially making this giant change the night before the competition. The problem was that the desk for the CBS show was set up in the beer garden, the same area where the Yelawolf show was supposed to go down. In the hour that Yelawolf was supposed to perform, they needed to film the CBS piece, and they couldn't do it with Yelawolf's playing in the background.

Justin had a few solutions—some really bad, some decent—but I didn't like any of them. While we were talking, Yelawolf was actually in the beer garden getting ready for his sound check. We had Tim Chan go out there and ask him and his team if we could move the show back an hour. Tim returned and said they basically said no. Apparently the request didn't go over well. We looked at other scheduling options, but moving the show to the end of the day was the best, so we told Tim to tell Yelawolf we needed him to move back an hour. He eventually agreed, but we had to pay for shipping on some stuff and cover some extra nights in a hotel for some team members. No big deal. I would later learn from the WME Entertainment contact who helped set the show up that changing the show time is the last thing to do. Apparently performers hate switching times, especially at the last minute.

We made the change, modified the schedule and everything was OK. But I was fuming about having to deal with this on Friday night. How could Justin, broadcast or someone from our team not have foreseen that problem earlier when we created the schedule?

We ended our meeting on a good note with positive spirits. I told the team, *"Two more days. Just make sure everything you are responsible for is always going smoothly. Do your job and we'll be fine."* We left happy, but I went home discouraged and beaten. I needed to sleep on it, wake up and shake the feeling because we still had two big days left.

*Day 3 of the Games—Saturday, Aug. 5*

## 2017 CROSSFIT GAMES TEAM EVENT 7: DRAG & DRIVE

### 150-FT. SKINNY BOB PULL

### 150-FT. SKINNY BOB PUSH

Saturday morning, the teams started the Bob event at 8 a.m. We didn't finalize this event until earlier in the week because we didn't have a Big Bob at Yarrow—actually, the sled was called the Skinny Bob. I changed the name because these sleds were narrower than the ones we typically use. We had the Demo Team play with a ton of variations, but we ended up having the teams pull the sled once down the field and push it once down the field—one continuous effort. We had pulled the Bob before, but never by its handles; we used a rope or two ropes.

This test was going to be simple and straightforward, so I decided to brief the teams that morning on the field and give them minimal rest before starting. They were on the field at 7:30, and I introduced the event. We had the Demo Team do the whole thing, pull 150 feet down and push 150 feet back. We ended up calling this test Drag & Drive, although I now think *"pull and push"* would have been better.

The fastest team was Functional Strength CrossFit, with a time of 1:23. Wasatch was at 1:30 for fifth, and CrossFit Mayhem finished in 1:35 for 12th.

The event was fast and brutal, and the athletes' legs were fried. I was very happy with the simplicity: down and back. No gimmicks, no special pieces. Just make it work. And I was very happy with the bodies on the floor after they finished. You had to push yourself to the absolute limit to get a top time. The slowest time was 2:01.

That event ended at 8:40, and we had 20 minutes to clear the gear and set up Strongman's Fear. Jobst Olschewski, our lead for the team on the soccer field and the gear crew, did a great job and got everything in place with time remaining.

### 2017 CROSSFIT GAMES EVENT 8: STRONGMAN'S FEAR

### MOVE YOKE, FARMERS LOG AND SLED 150 FT. ACROSS THE FIELD

### HANDSTAND WALK WHEN MOVING BACK

### M: 500-LB. YOKE, 200-LB. LOGS, 400-LB. SLED

### F: 340-LB. YOKE, 120-LB. LOGS, 310-LB. SLED

Right before the event started, I noticed something I didn't like: the loading of the carabiners. Carabiners were used to connect the straps for the sled to the webbing the athletes pulled on, and they were in a position where they could experience serious triaxial loading. Carabiners are meant to be loaded in the long direction, from the top to the bottom. Triaxial loading—loading in three directions—can lead to carabiner failure. It's not highly likely, but there's a chance it could happen. In the Navy, I was an avid rock climber and big into rope rescue techniques and systems. Before

CrossFit, that was my passion. So I had Bill and his team tape up the webbing to prevent triaxial loading.

The actual event—including the changes we had made a few days prior—was good. I would have preferred it to be a tad longer, but we had shortened the handstand walk, so the faster times made sense.

We let them select the order of objects they carried, and it was not always easy to follow the event. As a spectator, it was sometimes hard to tell how many items someone had moved. But this way was still far better than the original plan.

On the male side, the farmers handles ended up being a challenge for some of the lighter males. For the most part, the items were about the right weight. We had determined the loads in on-site testing during Games week. We tested the event a handful of times on Wednesday before the Games started, and then we tested one last time in the morning before the event.

The final male heat saw an epic battle for first. Mat looked like he was going to take the win, but Fikowski came across the line at about the same time and was able to sprint through the line to finish 9 hundredths of a second ahead of Mat to take the heat and the overall victory with a time of 4:13.22. Mat's time was 4:13.31. Their race to the finish is probably going to be considered one of the epic moments of the Games.

Jeff Patzer and Dakota Rager, both smaller guys, were the only two men to hit the time cap.

On the women's side, Katrin ended up crushing the event with a solid time of 3:55. The second-place athlete wasn't close: It was Tennil Reed-Beuerlein with a time of 4:17. No women hit the cap.

To create a better visual, I think I should have fixed the order of the stuff you had to carry across. That way you could really tell who was winning. But this version allowed for strategy and thought, which is important. I really liked that. Overall, I thought the test was great and the visual was OK. I felt good with the event—not blown away but happy.

We had a 50-minute break to transition from the north lot to the Coliseum, where the athletes were greeted by numerous barbells.

## 2017 CROSSFIT GAMES EVENT 9: MUSCLE-UP CLEAN LADDER

8 ROUNDS OF:

4 BAR MUSCLE-UPS

2 CLEANS, ASCENDING WEIGHT

M: 225-245-265-285-305-320-335-350 LB.

F: 145-160-175-190-205-215-225-235 LB.

I was very pleased with this event. We used 80 bars of various weights, and we used different colored bars. To help spectators follow the event, the bars were laid lengthwise on the floor. When an athlete approached a bar, he or she had to rotate it to be perpendicular with the lane before performing the clean. The big twist the athletes learned in their briefing that day was that the bar muscle-ups would be singles. Both aspects worked out great. Turning the barbells allowed you to see how far someone had advanced, and the multiple muscle-up bars were enough of a change to make the athletes reconsider how hard they would push. Cody Anderson had a very unique way of attacking them in the early stages of the test. He would perform a muscle-up, swing off with a really large leap and land on the ground, where he instantly rebounded and jumped up into the next bar muscle-up. It was very efficient and fast, but as the weights got heavier and he slowed up, he abandoned the technique.

During the first heat, I noticed the stagger we had created with the bars for safety caused the floor to look very confusing. We had staggered bars laid all across the floor, with no clear separation between them, so I had the signage team run lengths of red tape on the floor to isolate the sections by weight. They did this between the first and second men's heats and had to work fast to make the floor more understandable for the fans, athletes and viewers at home. I wish we had done that before the event. But that's a learning opportunity, and everyone on the team will grow as a result.

This event starts slowly but gets very exciting within minutes. Once athletes get to the bars in the 300s, you quickly see who's going to finish and who is not. Nineteen male athletes finished it—about exactly what I had predicted. I had planned for 50 percent of the athletes to finish, and I had played with lots of different loading schemes based on the clean numbers of the athletes in the field. Testing with people such as Julian Alcaraz, Lindsey Valenzuela and members of the Demo Team really helped me tie it together.

On the women's side, I went with slightly heavier weights than normal because it seems like we usually make the women's weights a little too light. As a result, only nine women beat the cap. The women's weight was a little too aggressive: I would have liked to have seen about 50 percent of them finish.

Back to the men's competition. One of the highlights of this event was Cody Anderson's fight to lift the 350-lb. barbell twice to finish the event. He missed one of the cleans at that weight, regrouped and then hit it. Cody weighs 170 lb., so it was a double-body-weight clean twice. I think it was even a PR, but I'm not sure.

Mat ended up crushing his heat and finishing with a time of 7:40. In that same heat, Alex Anderson and Scott Panchik were not too far behind. Alex finished at 7:58, and Scott finished at 8:05. Scott was slowly climbing back up the leaderboard. Ben Smith was fourth with a time of 8:09.

Most of the athletes did singles, but I remember seeing Travis Mayer doing touch-and-go reps all the way up to 300. I like when people do things like that to put on a good show for the crowd and essentially show off their strengths. In the end, he finished seventh. Who knows? Maybe if he had done singles he could have pushed a little harder and gone faster. Of note, Brent Fikowski couldn't finish the last bar. He got capped and took 22nd. That's a big swing from taking third in the snatch event the day before. On the same note, it was quite surprising to see EZ Muhammad hit the time cap given how much barbell work he does and how he swears by the Olympic lifts.

On the female side, I was really surprised to see Brooke Wells cap. She was 14th. To me, this event should be considered to play to her strengths. She's good at bar muscle-ups, but in this test, they're really an afterthought. She's always great at the lifts. In Squat Clean Pyramid at the 2016 Games, she finished fourth. Her 14th-place finish here, combined with her performance on the snatch, makes me wonder if she came in too lean and too light. You always want to train your weaknesses, but that should not negatively affect your traditional strengths. On the same note, Katrin also capped in this event, placing 24th. Again, that's interesting to me because I've always considered her strong enough for events like this.

This event was all Tia-Clair. She crushed it in 7:12. Her nearest competitor was Kara, who finished second in 7:55. When Tia finished, I leaned over to Sevan, who was standing behind me, and said, *"She just won the Games."*

*"Really?"*

*"Yup,"* I said. *"This is the moment she won the Games."*

It obviously ended up being more complicated than that, and more factors affected everything, but at that moment I knew Tia was going to win.

I was very happy with how this event looked and played out. I think we could have gone a tad lighter on the women's side, but I'm not too worried about that. The event looked great, the races were fun to watch, and the athletes who would soon be crowned the Fittest on Earth won the event.

After the individuals, we had two Team events to knock out. I remember it was a clusterfuck to swap those 80 bars for the Team gear. Well, it was more like controlled chaos. The transition went well, but it took all the time we had. We went right up to the wire setting the next event up, but we made it.

2017 CROSSFIT GAMES TEAM EVENT 8: COUPLE COUPLETS

AS PAIRS COMPLETE:

16-20-24 SYNCHRO BAR MUSCLE-UPS

50 GHD SIT-UPS

THEN, 2 ROUNDS OF:

15/10-CAL. ASSAULT BIKE

8-10-12 REPS OF PARTNER DEADLIFTS (545 LB.)

I was happy with how this event played out. It wasn't the easiest to follow in the beginning, but by the end you could really tell who was winning and where everyone was. It looked horrible in terms of its effects on the athletes—as so many of the Team events did this year.

For the first couplet, teams had a few options: They could set the pairs any way they wanted and select which pair would do which set of bar muscle-ups. I was really surprised to see a few teams use mixed pairs on the set of 24. I figured the best strategy was to use two men for that set, but I guess some females were better at muscle-ups than two of the men on their teams. If they weren't, those teams made a huge mistake.

In the first heat or so, I didn't see many teams finish, and I was a little worried. But more teams finished in the later heats. Overall, 15 teams finished under the time cap. That was fine for me. I didn't have great expectations that all teams would finish, but I wanted at least the top teams to do so. And that happened. The fastest team was Wasatch, who crushed it in a time of 16:23. I remember watching Mayhem fight to catch up, but they couldn't close the gap. They took second in 17:19. For all its moving parts, this event worked out well.

We had another crazy transition to set up for the next Team event, Worm Rotation. We were able to get the gear switched out in time, but we weren't able to program this one so many teams could finish.

2017 CROSSFIT GAMES TEAM EVENT 9: WORM ROTATION

AS MF PAIRS:

40 PULL-UPS OR 30 T2B OR 18/13-CAL. SKIERG

17 WORM CLEANS AS A TEAM

40 PULL-UPS OR 30 T2B OR 18/13-CAL. SKIERG

15 WORM CLEANS AS A TEAM

40 PULL-UPS OR 30 T2B OR 18/13-CAL. SKIERG

13 WORM CLEANS AS A TEAM

EACH ROUND, PAIRS COMPLETE A DIFFERENT EXERCISE

Only three teams finished. Ouch. That wasn't my plan. Late in the game, I had upped the reps from the version my testing team had performed, and that change moved this event into the unfinishable realm for most teams. Wasatch finished in 9:19, CrossFit Mayhem was second in 9:32, and CrossFit OC3 took third in 9:52. I should have reduced the reps on the cleans to ensure more teams could finish, but I missed that. Sadly, this wasn't the only event in which my time cap was too aggressive.

After this event, we had a break. I brought out the Individual athletes and briefed them on the final event of the night: Heavy 17.5. They were all excited, as were the fans. It's a great test, and it was going to be amazing to see all these athletes do it with heavier loads. The women would be doing thrusters with 95 lb.—the load men used in the Open.

### 2017 CROSSFIT GAMES EVENT 10: HEAVY 17.5

### 10 ROUNDS OF:

### 9 THRUSTERS (135/95 LB.)

### 35 DOUBLE-UNDERS

While this event was being set up, I went back to see the athletes. They were all excited and also very nervous. Most didn't know how to strategize for this one. Some were talking about breaking it up. Having seen our testers do it, I knew you couldn't break it up. But I didn't share that info.

The men were first up, and the floor looked amazing: 10 bars per lane, 100 bars on the floor. Josh Bridges was in the first heat. He was having a rough Games, so this was his chance to shine—and that he did. He flew through the event in 8:41, which would end up being the second-fastest time overall. As he usually is, Josh was pumped when he finished, and the fans loved it, too.

On this event, you could quickly see the spread and who was winning. Even on Muscle-Up Clean Ladder, it was not as easy to view. In that event, athletes moved back to the rig, so there were times when the race was not as clear as I would have liked. But on this event, athletes just moved forward, so it was clear as day who was thriving and who was struggling.

On the male side, only Alec Smith capped at the 12-minute mark. I don't know what was going on with him, and I was kinda surprised that he capped. What was not surprising was Mat's performance in the final heat. He crushed those in his heat and was closely watching the clock to make sure he got the top time overall. He ended up finishing in 8:24, 17 seconds faster than Josh. These times were incredible.

What the women did was—arguably—more impressive. Only two athletes capped: Alexis Johnson and Casey Campbell. Here's the impressive part: 18 women went sub 10. Eighteen women posted times that would have placed them in the 95th percentile of men in Workout 17.5 in the Open. And eight women went sub 9: Katrin Davidsdottir, Brooke Wells, Carol-Ann Reason-Thibault, Sam Briggs, Kari Pearce, Kristin Holte, Tia-Clair Toomey and Kara Webb. Tia finished second with a time of 8:01, and Kara went sub 8. Her time was 7:53. Some men who went to Regionals this year did not score 7:53 on 17.5 with the same weight.

Leading into the Games, I was really excited about this event, and it didn't disappoint. I was very pleased with this one. I was very happy with Saturday for the most part. This day ended great, the energy was high, the event was great, and we had some good momentum going forward. I was, for once during these Games, happy.

We closed the event off with our nightly meeting while Yelawolf was performing in the beer garden. Once our meeting was done, I walked out to see him, and I heard the crowd chanting, *"Yelawolf, Yelawolf!"* Yelawolf wasn't even out there. He had been in his green room for the last 10 minutes, but the excited fans were chanting for an encore. He didn't do one, but I'm happy the fans liked it.

I went back to my hotel in a good place, in a good state of mind. One more day. Everything was on track and going great.

Tomorrow morning would change all of that.

*Day 4 of the Games—Sunday, Aug. 6*
Sunday: The final day of the CrossFit Games.

I woke up early and I had a text from Boz that said the hay bales were really high and we needed to test Madison Triplet. I told him to rally the Demo Team and get them to test it out. That was put in motion while I was getting ready, and I didn't think I'd be able to get there in time to see it. Luckily, I showed up as they were getting warmed up.

Apparently hay bales are not the same everywhere. They didn't even have hay bales similar to the size of the ones we had in California, so we had to play with some other options. They had really gigantic blocks that might work, so we checked one out and then signed off on it. The bales were delivered the day before the event, so we couldn't do any testing. Once we got them set up, we realized how big they actually were.

Because the bales of hay—straw, actually—were so big, the thought was that we needed to drop the reps a little, from 9 to 7. We did the right thing and had it tested. On Sunday morning. A few hours before the event.

A few of members of the Demo Team tested a 7-rep version, and Alex Parker did a 9-rep version at the same time. After a few rounds, it became clear that the 9-rep version would be too lengthy, so we changed it to 7 reps for both men and women.

The cool thing was that the five rows of straw looked great. The event looked epic and grand in scale. I was thrilled with how the visual turned out.

After we figured all this out, I had some time before the competition kicked off. At the Affiliate Lounge—which was a huge hit—Coach Glassman was speaking to the Brazilian affiliate owners who were at the Games. I decided to go over there for a minute and listen to him. They seemed engaged and were asking questions about the Games, such as if they're ever coming to Brazil. *"Maybe one year, but not in the near future,"* I answered in my head.

After listening to Greg for a few minutes, I went back to my trailer in the Rogue area. I hung out there for a few minutes and walked out to find Bill. Bill found me instead. I had a guest with me to introduce to him, but Bill had a sense of urgency I don't often see from him.

*"Dave, we need to talk."*

I politely excused our guest because I could tell by Bill's voice that something was wrong. I asked him what was going on, and he told me the weight on the bars in Heavy 17.5 last night was off by 10 lb. All the weights were wrong.

For a minute, I felt like I was in a dream.

*"This can't be happening,"* I thought. It felt surreal. But then I quickly snapped out of that and asked him if all the bars were consistent. He said yes, the error was consistent. Every male had used 125 lb. and every female had used 85 lb.

I actually smiled. The error sucked. It ruined the perfect story I was looking for with that event, but it didn't affect the actual test. The test was still equal for all athletes.

"OK. It's fine. We'll move on, and I'll take a moment to think about how we handle it," I told Bill.

At this point, I was very level. Nothing could be done. No need to blow up or get angry. It had happened, and it had happened 12 hours ago. We just needed to decide how to handle it. I called Justin over, and we discussed the next steps. We both agreed we needed to admit the error and make a public statement, so we had our team draft up an announcement, and we showed it to Bill. Within the hour, we announced the mistake on our website, so it was public. Our social-media team asked if they were supposed to put the announcement out in their channels, and I told them not to: Just keep it on the site and let it spread via that outlet. We did our part. We didn't hide anything, and we didn't try to cover anything up. A mistake was made. And we owned it.

Bill was devastated. He apologized profusely. Ultimately, his team was responsible for providing the correct bars. I don't blame Bill, though. I blame my team. I'm disappointed in myself, even. There are so many details I see and look for, and I catch a lot. I have a really good eye for noticing things. I didn't look at the bars. I didn't verify them. I feel like I should have, but in the same sense I also realize I shouldn't have to. I have people and teams to do that. Boz is in charge of the Individual competition, so he's responsible, too. Chris Smith had the floor in the Coliseum, so he bears some responsibility, too. Stephane, head of competition, is also responsible. Basically there are three to five people in the system who didn't do part of their job and failed.

One thing I know for certain: It won't happen again. We will all learn from this and understand how to correct the issue. Something tells me this never would have happened in Carson. I almost want to blame it on the new venue and the new working environment. Something like this needed to happen here, and we got it out of the way.

One of the big stories of Heavy 17.5 was the comparison between the women at the Games and the men like me who used the same weight in the Open. I wanted people to be wowed when comparing their times with those of the women. Basically, we lose that effect because of this error. It happened on the test where it mattered most. That's the funniest part to me. This error could have happened in numerous other events, but it happened in the one where the weight was the story.

Bill said a volunteer on the Rogue team noticed the error after the event was over. The volunteer noticed that a bar from the event was a 25-pounder, not a 35-pounder. That's how the big mistake was made. Rogue has a ton of short specialty bars we use at the Games. Those bars are not very common—they are only seen in our competitions. And if you have two or three sets of bars that are within 10 lb. of each other and not perfectly, clearly marked, an error could be made. Considering all this, it's not hard to imagine how the mistake happened.

It was not a great way to start Sunday, but I had to let that one roll off my shoulders quickly. We had a full day of competition to get to.

### 2017 CROSSFIT GAMES EVENT II: MADISON TRIPLET

5 ROUNDS OF:

RUN 450 M

7 HAY-BALE CLEAN BURPEES

M: 100-LB. SANDBAG F: 70-LB. SANDBAG

On the men's side, Ricky Garard took first in 15:48. He had impressed me all weekend. He's legit and will be competitive for years to come. Vellner took second and Mat took third. Ricky's winning time was about 40 seconds faster than Vellner's second-place time. Fikowski was fourth. The eventual podium finishers were in the top four in Madison Triplet.

Josh was 19th on this event—another surprise to me. I expected him to do much better than that. Other low finishes on the male side included Ben Smith (25th), Noah Ohlsen (26th) and Scott Panchik (30th). Going into this event, Noah was poised to be on the podium for the first time in his career. This event was the start of a slide that would continue and dash those hopes.

On the female side, Sam Briggs won, followed by Kristin Holte and Tia-Clair Toomey. Kara Webb was ninth with a time of 18:27. Chyna Cho was just in front of her in eighth, and Alessandra Pichelli took seventh. I was surprised to see Kara and Alessandra in the top 10 because running events have typically not played to their strengths. Kara was 5 seconds behind Alessandra. Had Kara pushed a little harder and jumped two places, she would have won the Games. Of course, you can play this Game all over the leaderboard and *what if?* the hell out of it. I chose to do it here because this is Sunday, the final day of competition, and there is only one more event before the final.

Katrin's 13th-place finish was a surprise to me, too. I expected more from her on an event in which running was the dominant feature. But the biggest surprise was Sara Sigmundsdottir's 22nd-place finish.

Eleven women were capped in this event. No men hit the cap. In hindsight, I would have made this event a little longer for the men. I should have kept the men's reps at 9 and scaled the women to 7. I think the timing for the women was right. I liked the movements and the clean weights—super light, just to keep them going. Overall, I was happy with how this one played out. It was a good start to Sunday after a really bad start to Sunday.

2017 CROSSFIT GAMES TEAM EVENT 10: BURPEE LITTER

3 ROUNDS, AS TRIOS, WITH BODY ARMOR, OF:

250-M LITTER RUN

18 HAY-BALE BURPEES

M: 20-LB. VEST F: 14-LB. VEST

ORDER: MMM AND FFF TRIOS

In this one, the timing for the women's work and men's work was close but not spot on. We should have programmed different reps for each sex, but I realized that once the event was in full swing. I pulled Todd Widman and Chuck Carswell to the side to tell them that.

This event had a lot of moving parts, and after seeing the first heat go off fine, I left for the Coliseum to rehearse the announcement of the interval event with the Demo Team and the crew that was setting it up.

The setup looked amazing. The ropes made it look as if you were climbing to the ceiling.

We went over a few items and spent some time talking about the timing. Then I went back out to the north lot to watch the last heat of the Team competition.

The final heat featured a close race between Mayhem and Wasatch. Wasatch was winning most of the time, with Mayhem right on their heels. On the final lap, I saw the three men from Mayhem coming in behind the Wasatch trio, and toward the end of the run the Mayhem men made a last-minute switch to put Rich on the litter. Yards away from the transition point, they made a final switch. The two exchanges were literally about 30 yards apart. As soon as the men got back to their team, they took off for the finish line, but Rich sprinted ahead of everybody else. He was his own man on his own mission. He passed the Wasatch team, which was, for the most part, running together. Rich crossed the line to stop the clock at 14:39, and Wasatch clocked in at 14:40.

It looked like some members of the Wasatch team were actually ahead of Rich, and most of the team was definitely in front of the other Mayhem athletes. But, Rich played this game right. In years past, we had said the time stops when the whole team crosses the finish line—the athlete wearing the chip has to be the last one in the group. That rule is so hard to enforce in the heat of the moment. So at Regionals this year we made a change: Time stops when the chip crosses the line. That means you could send the athlete with the chip first or last. It was all up to the teams. That being the rule, Rich and Mayhem adjusted their strategy and took advantage of the rule to win.

I was near the finish line, and I saw Adrian Conway shaking his head in disapproval. He and Rich were having some words—nothing bad, just going back and forth on it. As I was approaching, I heard Rich say, "*Yeah, the rule's stupid.*" But he was very familiar with the rule and the game, and he took advantage of it.

I walked up and congratulated Rich. I said something to Adrian, and he tried pushing back on the win. I was like, "*Hey, they gamed it properly. Good on them.*"

The finish was great, but what's funny is that neither team had the best time. The top time was 13:58, posted in an earlier heat by CrossFit JST, which went on to finish 15th overall in the Games. It was impressive that their time was almost a minute faster than those of the top two teams overall.

During the 45-minute break that followed the Team event, I took the individuals into the stadium and briefed them on 2223 Intervals.

2017 CROSSFIT GAMES EVENT 12: 2223 INTERVALS

3 2-MINUTE ROUNDS AND 1 3-MINUTE ROUND OF:

2 ROPE CLIMBS

10/7-CAL. SKIERG

MAX-REP OHS (155/105 LB.)

REST 1 MINUTE

GO UNTIL 75 REPS OF OHS ARE COMPLETE

The athletes all seemed to be excited for this one, and Katrin asked me what happens if you finish all the reps before the fourth round. I explained what would happen and told them how unlikely that scenario would be. After that conversation, apparently Katrin and a few other athletes talked about how they would finish the 75 reps in 3 rounds and not need the fourth.

I was really interested to see this one play out: This was the first time we did an interval event like this with the same buy-in work in each round. In creation, this one went through a ton of revisions and testing, and I was very worried about getting the reps and the weight right. I also adjusted the time domains in testing. In the beginning, it was four 2-minute rounds of work, with 1 minute of rest between each round. When looking at the schedule, I realized we could make the final round 3 minutes—2-2-2-3, with 1 minute of rest between rounds. This adjustment would allow athletes to finish all the overhead squats. Had we not made that change, two males would have finished (*Mat and Travis Williams*) and 4 females would have finished (*Katrin, Annie, Kristin and Kara*). With the format we used, 11 men and 16 women finished. These numbers are much better. I was very happy with just that change. Toward the end of the weekend, it's better to see more people finish an event like this.

The event itself starts out slow. The first 2 rounds are about getting work done and establishing position. By the third and fourth round, it's obvious who's winning and who's getting crushed. Our floor plan for this beautifully showcased the race, and rounds 3 and 4 were exciting because you saw who was close to finishing and who was not. After a few large chunks of stationary squatting in the beginning, we had the athletes advance their barbells every 3 reps to really show who was where.

I think Katrin ended up doing 31 reps in her first round, and then on her second I think she did 23 or 24. Maybe less. But at that point I kinda knew she wouldn't hit 75 in 3 rounds. She was close—very close—but I think she ended up with 6-8 reps to do in the final set. She had the fastest time overall by about 18 seconds. Tia took 14th. I was surprised to see Tia so far back.

During the final heat, Kara was moving down the floor and nearing the finish line. After a certain point, we had athletes move forward every 3 reps. The final 3 reps—reps 73, 74 and 75—were to be done on a mat that had a red number 75 on it. The mat signified that's where the final 3 reps were to be performed. Before that, a mat with a white 72 on it indicated where athletes were to perform reps 70, 71 and 72. Kara was on this mat and finished her 72nd rep. She motioned to advance, and the judge nodded, so she ran and crossed the finish line without performing the last 3 reps. People instantly realized a mistake had been made. It was a mistake on her part as an athlete, but, more importantly, it was a mistake by our judge.

Our team got together and discussed a plan of action. Boz reviewed the film and figured out how long it took her to do 3 reps. We then decided to add that amount of time to her total time. It wasn't an ideal fix, but it was the best we could do in this situation. Boz let her know we were going to adjust her time because of the error, and she was fine with it. She was moved to fourth place.

As long as humans judge movement in this sport, there will always be mistakes. That is not an excuse, but it is a reality. If you watch an NBA or NFL game, officials regularly make the wrong calls. Sometimes judges make mistakes at the Games. Humans simply make mistakes. I understand this, and we take every precaution we can in training and preparing these judges for their roles, so these situations don't get me too riled up anymore. I just let it flow and didn't have much to say to the judge who made the error.

On the male side, Travis Williams set the time to beat in an early heat: 10:58. But we still had to see Mat attack this, and he's known for his superb positioning and strength in movements such as the thruster and overhead squat. Mat won his heat and the event in 10:54. The lowest score went to Noah Ohlsen. At one point, I saw him fall from the rope and struggle to get the second rope climb of his third or final set. I remember he started out with the fastest pace in Round 1. He crushed it, then started falling back, then had his meltdown. Going into Sunday, he had a podium place locked up. On Sunday's first two events, he took 26th and 38th. His podium hopes were slipping away.

I was very pleased with this test and this format. I think the movements were well chosen, and the timing and rep scheme worked to make it a great test and event. This format has a lot of potential to make a return to the Games. Probably not Regionals. But the Games for sure.

We had a break to set up the Team final, which I had announced to the athletes earlier in the day in their warm-up area. During the transition period, I announced the final event for the individuals: the Fibonacci Final. I briefed the male version first, and I had Albert-Dominic Larouche do it. He basically went through the whole thing. I didn't time him, but I think he finished under 6 minutes. He had done it a few days ago in testing and was in the mid-4s. I then told the women their final would have a different rep scheme. A couple of women actually expressed interest in having the same scheme as the men, but I said, *"Trust me. As is, it's fine."*

After that they all walked off the floor, and we scrambled to get it laid out for the Team final.

*Tuesday, Aug. 29, 4:27 p.m.*
It's been a little while since I've written anything. At this stage, I only have to talk about the final afternoon of the Games, but I haven't prioritized doing that in recent days. I wasn't even planning on writing today, but I'm forced to do so, and I'll step out of the chronology of events for a moment.

This afternoon, I received a note from our testing team: We had a couple of tests from the Games come back positive. A masters athlete, Tony Turski, second in the 55-59 division, tested positive for anastrolzole.

From Wikipedia: *"Some athletes and body builders use anastrozole as part of their steroid cycle to reduce and prevent symptoms of excess estrogen—gynecomastia, emotional lability and water retention."*

But more surprising and troubling was finding out that our third-place Individual finisher, Ricky Garard from Australia, failed his drug test, too. I'm disappointed by that because I actually like the kid and liked what I saw in him at the Games. He had a competitive fire in him, and I thought we would see him on the podium for years to come.

Garard had an elevated T/E ratio *(testosterone to epitestosterone)*, and he also tested positive for RAD140 *(classified as an anabolic agent known as a SARM, or selective androgen receptor modulator)* and GW1516 *(classified under hormone and metabolic modulators)*.

According to USADA.org, SARMS are *"a class of therapeutic compounds that have similar properties to anabolic agents, but with reduced androgenic properties. This property allows SARMs the advantage of androgen-receptor specificity, tissue selectivity, and the lack of steroid-related side effects."*

Also from USADA.org: *"Hormones and metabolic modulators are a group of substances that are not limited to hormones themselves. This group of substances often modifies how hormones work, either by blocking the action (of) a hormone or by increasing the activity of a hormone. There are many substances that fall into the category of 'Hormone or Metabolic Modulator.' ... Substances that activate AMP-activated protein kinases, for example AICAR, show promise in protecting cells against oxidative damage during stroke or in certain diseases like diabetes. Similarly, substances that activate peroxisome proliferator activated receptor modulators (PPARs) like GW1516, GW0742, L1655041 are experimental drugs under study to treat diabetes, lipid disorders and metabolic syndrome. AMP-activated protein kinases and PPARs are experimental drugs with no approved medical use at this time. However, these substances are synthesized by clandestine laboratories around the world but are still not approved for human use."*

We're still waiting on some test results to come back. I hope nobody else fails—especially individuals who are on the podium.

I'm not naive. I believe some people in our sport cheat and use chemical advantages to take them further in the sport at multiple levels. Some Games athletes cheat, but I believe they are few in number, largely because we test the athletes at this level so often. Some Regionals athletes cheat, and I think the number of people using at this level is probably higher than we expect—especially among those who place lowest at Regionals. And then there are all the other cheaters—people who don't make it to Regionals, people who aren't good enough to make it to the Games but compete in some of the big events that don't test. For whatever reasons, people choose to cheat—to gain a competitive edge, to see results faster, to look better.

But I also believe—and know—that of the top guys, more are clean than not. That includes guys such as Rich Froning, whom we have routinely tested at random times throughout the year. And it includes other winners. Until now, we have never had a Games podium finisher fail a test. It's disappointing.

It will still be a few weeks before we announce the failed test because of all the steps we have to go through with the testing agency and with Ricky. I think this will get a lot of attention when it comes out. People who say everyone in our sport is guilty will come out, make those accusations and bark louder than ever before. They will justify that because now they have their *"proof"*—someone popped. Of course, they will ignore the fact that the overwhelming majority of the field tested passed the test. But that won't matter.

I feel bad for the rest of the competitors because this positive test will potentially overshadow the hard work by the guys who are clean. Ultimately, positive tests make them look bad, too.

After all this, I can guarantee one thing: We are going to beef up our testing protocol. We already have a good system in place with Drug Free Sport. Obviously, it's working if we're catching a podium finisher at the Games. But I want to catch more guys or make it so cheaters are afraid to come to Regionals or the Games. I want to start testing more people at all stages of competition. I want to invest in a beefed-up program. And that's really what it comes down to: investment. We need to spend more on that program, and we will. This is a now big goal and priority for me for the remainder of 2017, and it will be a priority as we go into 2018.

Now I'll get back into the chronology of the CrossFit Games.

*Day 4 of the Games—Sunday, Aug. 6*
The teams only had one event remaining, and we only allowed the top 10 to do it. It's an event I spent a lot of time working with on paper and in testing. I went back and forth with different versions. The version I ended up using was stiff.

2017 CROSSFIT GAMES TEAM EVENT II: WORM COMPLEX

WHILE TEAM HOLDS WORM, PAIRS EACH PERFORM:

1 ROPE CLIMB

10 HANDSTAND PUSH-UPS

THEN, EACH PAIR PERFORMS:

2 ROPE CLIMBS

20 HANDSTAND PUSH-UPS

THEN, EACH PAIR PERFORMS:

3 ROPE CLIMBS

30 HANDSTAND PUSH-UPS

THEN, TEAM PERFORMS:

30 WORM COMPLEXES

WORM COMPLEX = I CLEAN, 2 SQUATS, DROP, STEP OVER

When they weren't working on rope climbs and HSPU, athletes were holding the lighter of the Worms we had, so they never had a true break. After the first section, they went to 30 Worm complexes: clean, squat, squat, drop, step over for 1 rep. Sadly, this event was over-programmed for the time cap, and only two teams finished. CrossFit OC3 won with a time of 23:58, and CrossFit Mayhem took second in 24:56. Wasatch tied for third, but they hit the time cap.

I would have liked at least half the field to finish, but I'm really happy that at least two finished. During the competition, I remember watching and thinking, *"Oh no, nobody is going to finish."* Thankfully, OC3 finished with about a minute remaining, and Mayhem completed the reps with a few seconds remaining.

I won't forget these lessons on the time caps and the programming. I always need to determine how aggressive I want to be with a time cap or if I have to reduce the reps, and we test to find the right numbers. In this case, the fault falls on me. But in terms of the test and the race, we accomplished what needed to be accomplished, and it was still a brutal test for the teams and an exciting race for the fans—a slow yet exciting race.

After the event, I walked over and announced Wasatch CrossFit as the 2017 Reebok CrossFit Games champions. They had had a great weekend. Their lowest overall placing was 26th in the men's half of the snatch event, but their next lowest placing was 11th. They were in the top 10 in everything else, and they finished first in four events.

Mayhem finished second. They never won a single event all weekend. They took second on the last four events and were able to claim the second spot on the podium. CrossFit Fort Vancouver finished third. They've been to the Games nine times in a row, which is a very impressive feat.

I've procrastinated in finishing this book. It's been about a week since my last entry, largely due to the Garard issue. I've avoided working on this as we decided internally how to handle everything. I let a few HQ people outside our core team know about the failed test, but not a lot of people. I still need to keep the information secure.

2017 CROSSFIT GAMES INDIVIDUAL EVENT 13: FIBONACCI FINAL

MEN

5-8-13 REPS OF:

HANDSTAND PUSH-UPS

KETTLEBELL DEADLIFTS (203 LB.)

THEN, 89-FT. KETTLEBELL OVERHEAD LUNGE (53-LB.)

WOMEN

3-5-8 REPS OF:

HANDSTAND PUSH-UPS

5-8-13 REPS OF:

KETTLEBELL DEADLIFTS (124 LB.)

THEN, 89-FT. KETTLEBELL OVERHEAD LUNGE (35-LB.)

The reduced rep scheme for the women was the right call. We ended up having 27 of 37 finish the event. I think if we had them do the same reps as the men, very few—if any—would have finished. The women did 10 fewer HSPU: We had 26 total for the men and 16 for the women. Notable athletes who struggled and didn't finish include Chyna Cho, Stacie Tovar and Margaux Alvarez. They are experienced athletes, so I was surprised to see them in that group.

Sara Sigmundsdottir was fastest, with a time of 3:13. That actually surprised me. A few years ago, she really struggled on the parallette handstand push-ups in a final event at the Games, so it was nice to see she had improved. That event win wouldn't be enough to put her on the podium. She hadn't done enough earlier in the weekend.

Annie Thorisdottir posted 3:18 as the second-fastest time, and Brooke Wells logged 3:28 in an earlier heat to take third. It was good to see Brooke finish strong. She had a tough Games this year.

Some have already started calling the race in the final heat the most exciting finish in the history of the CrossFit Games. Tia-Clair Toomey was only a few points ahead of Kara Webb going into the final. To win the Games, Tia had to finish in front of Kara—or if she finished behind her, she had to be very close without many people in between. Last year, I had watched Tia lose the Games on the final event to Katrin, and I was wondering if we were going to see her slip to second on this one. Kara had to beat Tia and have some people finish in between them for her to win the Games.

The two worked through the handstand push-ups and deadlifts, and Tia had a good lead over Kara. She wasn't winning the heat, but she only needed to be in front of Kara.

Tia made it to the lunges ahead of Kara. She got the kettlebells overhead and took off. This was the final part of the Games, essentially the victory lap as Tia won the CrossFit Games for the first time.

For a good stretch in the beginning, it looked like she was going to go unbroken, but then she put the kettlebells down. Kara, who had been slightly behind Tia, was marching to close the gap because Tia was resting. As the race between the two was playing out, other athletes were finishing, but all eyes were on the two Aussies.

They were less than 20 feet from the finish, lunging toward their own visions of CrossFit glory, with Tia slightly ahead.

At the last marker, a few feet from the finish line, Tia didn't lock out her final rep. She had to step back and do 2 more to finish, and Kara caught her.

The fans were losing their minds. It was probably the loudest crowd I've ever heard at one of our events. The energy and atmosphere were intense.

Tia crossed the finish line at the same time Kara was lunging past her. Almost together, they ran across the finish line and went to the floor exhausted.

It was too close to tell who finished ahead. If Tia had beaten Kara, Tia was the champion. If Kara had beaten Tia and people from other heats had finished in between them, Kara had a chance at victory.

It turned out that Kara crossed slightly ahead with a time of 3:47.80. Tia crossed right behind her with a time of 3:47.99. Luckily for Tia, nobody fell between them: Kara was seventh and Tia was eighth. From that finish, Tia won the CrossFit Games with 994 points, and Kara was second with 992. It was the closest finish, and yes, I can agree that it was the most exciting finish we've ever had for the female competition—and the male competition, too. We've never had an event that close for the men.

I was happy with how this test played out as a final event for the women. It was challenging, it was tough, and it was entertaining. The Fibonacci Final for the women was a great event that provided our most exciting finish ever, and I'm very happy about that.

In the men's version, we used 5-8-13 reps for both the handstand push-ups and the deadlifts. In testing, Julian had finished in about 4:30. At the Games, a few days before the event, we had Albert-Dominic Larouche do it, and he also completed it in 4:30 or so. Going into it, we were very confident men would finish—I thought at least 50 percent of the field or more. Man, was I wrong.

The first heat started, and as I watched them finish the deadlift/HSPU section, I slowly realized nobody in the first heat was going to finish. Not a single athlete. "*OK*," I thought. "*It's the first heat, the weakest of the field at this point. Surely in the next three heats someone will finish.*"

Then the second heat came and left with the same outcome. No one finished. And nobody was even close to finishing. I was really not in a good place at that point. This was not what I wanted to see. The set of 13 handstand push-ups was really taking the athletes a long time. Actually, even the set of 8 was slow, but by the time they got to the 13s, it was not looking good at all.

Finally, we had an athlete finish in the third heat: Logan Collins in 5:29. That was a great sign, I thought. If Collins could finish, then at least five or six men in the final heat would finish. And if six or seven athletes finished the event, I would be content.

As it turns out, nobody finished in the last heat. Fuck.

Mat was a few feet away from finishing, but he went very slowly on the event. He had an insurmountable lead in the overall standings, and he said later that he just wanted to meet the minimum work requirement and then chill. Once he did the minimum amount of work and was assured of the overall win, he realized he was basically winning his heat, so he decided to go for it. Had he been racing from the start, he surely would have finished, but that was not that case.

The buzzer signaled the time cap, and Mat was a few feet away from finishing. He continued through the line to stand on the finish platform. Everyone was very excited and cheering at the top of his or her lungs for him. It was his moment of victory, and he had won his heat even though he didn't finish.

For me, that moment was one of the lowest of the 2017 Games, and it haunted me for the rest of that evening and the days and weeks to come. I plan and rehearse these events, and I have athletes test them over and over so I know the events will accomplish what I want to accomplish. I feel like I missed the mark at the worst possible place: the final men's event of the Games.

Looking back, we should have made the time cap 7 minutes, not 6. Then a number of athletes would have finished. But from our testing sessions, it didn't really seem like a 7-minute cap was necessary. And almost always, the athletes at the Games are much faster than our testers, even in final events at the end of a long weekend of competition. This one haunted me for weeks.

Overall, the finish wasn't a stain on the event or the competition. Actually, hardly anyone noticed it or talked about it, partly because Mat had been so dominant, and partly because the women had provided such an epic finish. It was almost like people weren't expecting much more from the men's side. I was, though.

*Tuesday, Sept. 5, 10:46 a.m.*

I learned a lot from the 2017 Games and the time I spent constructing the event. It feels great to have the opportunity to learn from the process even in my 11th year of programming the Games.

The 2017 events were probably the most difficult and time consuming of all the tests I've ever programmed because of a variety of factors that we had to deal with this year—the first time we ran the Games outside California.

The biggest challenge was adapting to the new venue in Madison. The second biggest obstacle was the new format, with the Team, Age Group and Individual competitions all essentially happening at the same time. Each competition presented additional challenges and opportunities to grow.

I don't imagine it will ever be easy to program the Games. Every year, I anticipate greater challenges that will continue to drive me forward and help me determine how we can push the athletes and the community to the next level.

The 2017 edition of the CrossFit Games was the best yet, but I'm already excited about next year. The Games only wrapped a month ago, but I've already moved on. I've started planning for 2018, and I've already put ideas to paper.

The 12th edition of the Games will once again raise the bar of the competition. The 2018 Games will demand more of the athletes than the athletes ever demand of themselves, and they will once again prove to be the only test in the world that truly determines the Fittest on Earth.

Be prepared for an epic test of fitness in 2018.

§

Made in the USA
Columbia, SC
06 December 2018